WORKING SYSTEMICALLY WITH FAMILIES

WORKING SYSTEMICALLY WITH FAMILIES

FORMULATION, INTERVENTION AND EVALUATION

By

Arlene Vetere

and

Rudi Dallos

Routledge
Taylor & Francis Group
LONDON AND NEW YORK

First published 2003 by Karnac Books Ltd.

2 Park Square, Milton Park, Abingdon, Oxfordshire OX14 4RN
52 Vanderbilt Avenue, New York, NY 10017

Routledge is an imprint of the Taylor & Francis Group, an informa business

First issued in hardback 2019

British Library Cataloguing in Publication Data

A C.I.P. record for this book is available from the British Library

ISBN: 978-1-85575-988-6 (pbk)
ISBN: 978-0-367-32989-1 (hbk)

Edited, designed, and produced by The Studio Publishing Services Ltd, Exeter EX4 8JN

CONTENTS

FOREWORD

This book reminded me of my experience of working with trainees on a Clinical Psychology training course. The trainees were enviably competent and self-confident in using the CBT model they were taught on the course. However, when they encountered serious obstacles in the form of clients whose style of interaction did not seem to fit with their model or when they became aware of the full range of complex issues surrounding the presenting problem, systemic thinking could come across as a "life saver". Its conceptual rigour in mapping complex systems, its framework for exploring multiple realities, and its helpfulness in addressing the position of the practitioner and challenging their certainties all came into their own. It created a way out of the impasses created by the all too tempting categories of "unsuitable client" or "incompetent professional" into a coherent and dynamic framework for understanding relational dilemmas. However, while this book will be an invaluable introduction to family systems theory and practice for clinical psychology training courses, plugging a gap that Vetere and Dallos have identified as one of their motives for writing it, its remit runs much wider. It will prove an invaluable companion for any professional working in the public services, whether systemically trained or not. It covers an impressive range of theory, practice and research and, as such, is firmly grounded both in the application to different client groups and in the necessity for most practitioners of integrating different therapeutic approaches.

It is hard to think of two authors more qualified to bring all these different elements together in one compact and readable volume. As clinical psychologists and systemic family therapists, loyal to the traditions of each discipline, Vetere and Dallos appear to wear their two hats effortlessly. They bring with them a combination of wide, even encyclopaedic, knowledge of the family systems field, theoretical rigour, impressive clarity and a strong sense of being grounded in the "realities" of clinical practice. They can, therefore, write with authority and credibility about these areas within which this book is likely to prove most valuable; the broader context of professional training and the context of the public services, especially the NHS, within a multi-cultural and inegalitarian society.

The riches in this book are perhaps three-fold.

Firstly, the authors' concern, and I would add, their passion, is with theoretical integration. While systemic therapy is an alternative treatment model, it is also utilized as a meta-theory which can encompass and engage with many perspectives simultaneously without losing intellectual rigour.

The integrated model which Vetere and Dallos provide has, at its heart, the idea of formulation, intervention and evaluation. The former invites practitioners to make a provisional, good-enough-for-now hypothesis about the relationship between problem and system, which is always held as temporary and contingent, and subject to feedback and review as new information emerges through the interaction between family and professionals.

This model goes right to the heart of the aesthetics of systemic practice in its constant movement between pragmatic engagement and epistemological reflection which, while difficult to achieve, is essential if we are to maintain ethical practice.

I would argue that Vetere and Dallos provide a good model of this process in their treatment of theoretical developments in the family systems field, always explaining the contexts within which new ideas evolve, and demonstrating how the process of feedback alerts practitioners to new contexts from which to critique and revise theory.

They attend meticulously to issues of gender and power imbalances, and they invite reflexivity by engaging the reader in exercises at the end of most chapters.

The second great strength of this book lies in its detailed elaboration of how systemic practice extends into different practice areas, including excellent chapters on working with alcoholism, eating disorders, learning disability and family violence. In each case the description is enriched by the inclusion of research findings and, in keeping with their integrated approach, by perspectives from different theoretical models.

The research chapter in particular is a model of clarity and I can confidently predict that it will become essential reading for a whole range of training courses, as will the summary of systemic perspectives on consultation.

Thirdly, the book demonstrates how systemic thinking and practice has achieved an excellent fit with the current preoccupations and priorities in the modern health and social services. These include effective inter-professional and inter-agency communication, involvement of and collaboration with service users, and flexibility of service delivery. In relation to evidence based practice, which can constitute a straightjacket for therapists, Vetere and Dallos demonstrate how, in their words, "formulation offers an enlightened perspective that enables a thorough consideration of what constitutes 'evidence'. Without this we may be subject to a diminished approach to 'evidence'".

In summary, this book constitutes another marker in the increasingly high profile of systemic therapy at so many levels of public service, and within a wide range of professional and therapeutic training programmes. Both of these authors have played a pivotal role over many years in these developments, and the publication of this book will notch up another debt we owe them.

Gwyn Daniel
Senior Clinical Lecturer and Systemic Psychotherapist,
Tavistock Clinic
Co-Director, Oxford Family Institute

ABOUT THE AUTHORS

Arlene Vetere taught a final year undergraduate option in Reading University Psychology Department on family process for ten years, during the 1990s. At the time, there were only a few like-minded colleagues in other psychology departments teaching similar courses. The difficulty always was, of course, that this option came in the final year, without the benefit of previous undergraduate teaching. Difficult, because the undergraduates were expected to grapple with complex theoretical, methodological, and ethical issues involved in the study of the family that are not found in the study of individuals.

Arlene trained as a clinical psychologist in the early 1980s, at a time when family therapy/systemic psychotherapy was not considered to be the proper activity of a clinical psychologist. She had to struggle to insist on a family therapy placement in her final year of training, which was generously provided by Andy Treacher.

Rudi Dallos works as a consultant clinical psychologist specializing in work with adolescents and their families, and as a clinical/academic tutor on the Plymouth Clinical Psychology Training Course. He has previously worked for the Open University and the SE Thames Clinical Psychology Training Course. His research and writing interests have been in the area of family therapy, family belief systems, and couples' dynamics. Rudi has published a significant number of peer-reviewed journal articles as well as several books relating to his research, teaching, and clinical experience, examples of which are, *Family Belief Systems, Couples' Sex and Power* (with S. Dallos), *Interacting Stories,* and *Introduction to Family Therapy* (with R. Draper). Dr Dallos participated in an EU-funded family therapy distance learning project in which he played a key role in writing the learning materials. He presents his work at national and European conferences on family therapy. Rudi has supervised a wide range of post-graduate research and is currently engaged in a research project exploring the links between attachments and family representations.

Introduction and overview

Why did we write this book?

In our view a systemic approach continues to offer a radical perspective on the understanding and treatment of human distress. This might seem surprising given that the original ideas were articulated half a century ago. However, it is the continued usefulness and adaptability of systemic ideas that sustains their value in our professional practice and personal lives.

Both of us work in multiple clinical and training contexts. In our clinical work we are required to work with individuals, couples, families and larger groups, teams and agencies across the life span. We find it helpful to draw on models and interventions, such as Cognitive Behaviour Therapy, Personal Construct Therapy, psychodynamic and attachment theory and narrative approaches, alongside systemic ideas. This can be seen as a form of eclecticism, which many colleagues appear to share. However, one of the golden threads of this book is that systemic theory can offer a framework for integrating diverse ideas. Systemic thinking offers a new way of seeing human problems and offers a coherent and dynamic framework in conceptualizing such problems. In offering a recursive approach to formulation, systemic thinking drives our approach to conceptual eclecticism.

The practice of formulation is central to many clinical disciplines. Alongside the growing interest in formulation there exists a parallel critique, that questions its value. For example, some narrative therapists argue that a position of curiosity and engagement can be diminished by practising formulation. For us, formulation offers a broad opportunity to conceptualize problems and solutions in collaboration with all participants in the therapeutic process. This can include thinking about problems from different levels and contexts of analysis, drawing together the different models in a clear and systematic way. So, for us there need not be any contradictions between using, for example, ideas from narrative approaches and formulation to guide practice. Thus, accountability for our practice lies not only in the theories we use, but in how we integrate those theories. We have heard it argued that sometimes it is hard to find the time to develop formulations. Though sympathetic to the demands on busy clinicians, we think all of us engage in this activity implicitly, if not explicitly. Therefore, taking on the practice of formulation as central to our thinking with clients about the work can help us stay open, accountable, and clear in our thinking—in short it can help expose our prejudices.

In our working culture of Evidence Based Practice (EBP) (DOH, 1996) we are increasingly asked to provide evidence of therapeutic effectiveness. Formulation offers an enlightened perspective that enables a thorough consideration of what constitutes "evidence". For example, by classifying and making explicit with our clients what we are doing together, and why, offers us all a broader and ecologically valid approach to "evidence". Without this, we may be subject to a diminished approach to clinical effectiveness. Taking a proactive position towards formulation in the current climate can help reduce the risk of the imposition of limited and inappropriate measures of clinical activity.

Neglecting families—the study of the family?

We might reasonably expect that the discipline of psychology might provide the well-spring for ideas to promote therapy with families and other relational groupings. Yet, unlike sociology, the discipline of psychology has paid scant attention in its history to the family. Rather, the focus in mainstream psychology has been on individual processes and, where the family has been considered, it is often seen as a context for individual development across the life span. Even social psychologists have been slow to realize the potential of the study of the family for the explication of group processes and intergroup relations. Developmental psychologists, whose main focus has long been mother–child or carer–child interactions, relatively recently have taken more interest in the study of sibling relationships (Brody, 1996), non-shared environments for child development (Plomin, 1986), and father–child relationships (Lamb & Billings, 1997), but still have a long way to go in thinking about household family groups as worthy of study in their own right.

Other social science and biological science disciplines have not been shy of studying family and kin groups, family processes and wider systems within which family groups inter-relate with other cultural systems. Sociology, anthropology, ethology, biology, and geography, as examples, have long histories of research and theorizing with family groups. However, where these disciplines could benefit from more exchange with psychology would be in the attempt to illuminate the inner emotional experiences of family life. And where these disciplines could benefit academic psychology would be in highlighting the importance of family study in its own right, not just as another context for the study of the individual.

There is no doubt that many psychological psychotherapies besides systemic psychotherapy have made the study of the interior of the family important to their practice; for example, group analytic psychotherapists, attachment theorists, and object relations therapists. But their approach has been largely informed by the need for clinical theorizing and clinical practice. The schools of psychotherapy have paid less attention to rigorous observational studies of family life that go beyond the parent–child relationship, or the couple relationship, and include larger group interaction with people not in receipt of clinical services.

Writing in 1987, Arlene Vetere and Tony Gale decried the apparent lack of academic interest in family groups within mainstream psychology. Neil Frude (1991) joined us in a clarion call to psychologists to undertake the study of the family in his book

Understanding Family Problems. Writing this present book, we can see little evidence that the situation has changed much. And this is a real pity, because if family psychology is not taught routinely to undergraduate psychologists, where does that leave clinical, counselling, and educational psychologists?

Applied psychology trainings have changed substantially in the intervening years. For example, clinical and counselling psychologists in training are now expected to be knowledgeable about systemic psychotherapy approaches, and to be systemic in their approach to case formulation. It is interesting to us that this expectation is not built on any general undergraduate training in family psychology. Thus, we think many clinical psychologists in training have not been well served in this regard by their first degree. And it is probably too much to expect busy doctoral clinical psychology training courses to teach family psychology at more than a cursory level. This becomes increasingly important when we consider the field of family psychology to be the academic base on which much of the theorizing in systemic psychotherapy is based. We hope this book will go some way towards filling the gaps for clinical and counselling psychologists, both qualified and in training.

The situation in North America is different. The American Psychological Association (APA) has had an active division of Family Psychology for over 20 years and not surprisingly much of the academic research and thinking has originated within the North American context. Writing and working in the UK, we wonder to what extent this large and vigorous body of research findings can be translated into our European context without questioning the cultural specificity of the findings. It seems to us that further study of the applicability of the North American research and the clinical thinking that flows from it must take place. And this brings us back to our first point—we need to equip our undergraduates and our post-graduates with the theories, methods and skills to observe, enquire and research the experience of family life.

Orientation of the book—the storyline

The structure of the book illustrates our approach to formulation, intervention, and evaluation. The book proposes that these three are linked as an interlocking triangle:

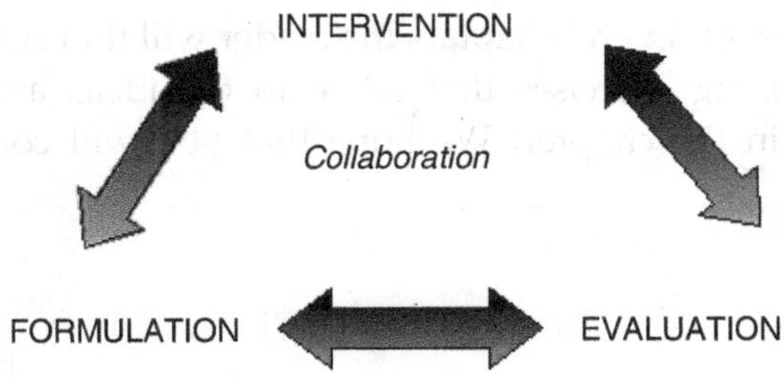

We suggest that guiding the relationship between each of these pairs: formulation-evaluation, formulation-intervention and evaluation-intervention is the concept of working collaboratively with families and others.

A brief outline of the contents

Chapters One and Two highlight some significant and enduring systemic ideas and their applications in systemic practice. This is summarized in terms of three suggested phases of theoretical development. A number of illustrative windows are used throughout to bring the ideas to life.

Chapter Three is a core chapter, which attempts to lay out a model of systemic formulation. It builds on Chapters One and Two, showing how systemic ideas and practices can be woven together within a coherent framework. It also makes explicit the processes involved in formulation that have evolved within systemic practice. Specifically, this chapter attempts to build on the influential approach to progressive hypothesizing developed by the Milan team.

Chapter Four reviews research into family therapy, process, and outcome as the empirical basis for family therapy and systemic practice. It links with the previous chapter in showing how clear formulation assists the research endeavour.

Some recent developments in theory and application are critically reviewed in Chapters Five and Six.

In the concluding chapter, which draws together formulation, intervention, and evaluation, we attempt to look into the future of systemic practice, especially in terms of our interlocking triangle.

At the end of several chapters the reader will find some reflexive notes containing exercises that relate to the ideas and processes introduced in the chapter. We hope that you will consider them helpful.

CHAPTER ONE

What is family therapy and systemic practice?

From the intra-psychic to the trans-personal

The central organizing thesis of the systemic paradigm is the focus on interpersonal relationships and the move to thinking about relationships as the cradle and web of human experience and development. For us, the excitement of this paradigm shift lies in understanding and explaining individual experiences in relational terms and in understanding individual processes in the context of emotionally significant relationships. Thus, individual distress can no longer be seen only as the product of the individual's psychology, but rather as a complex iterative process that is understood in terms of relational dynamics at many levels of contextual understanding. Applied psychologists' preference for (ongoing) formulation maps well on to systemic thinking, so that the particular circumstances of the people seeking our help will dictate how much relative importance is attached to individual, relational, group, cultural, and societal levels of explanation. Making the connections between these levels of explanation and their relationship over time, connecting past to present to future, is the powerful contribution that systemic thinking can make to psychotherapy formulation and ensuing practice. Thus, when we use the term "systemic", we are using it in the wider sense of its meaning as rooted in developments in family systems theories (Dallos & Urry, 1999; Vetere & Gale, 1987), rather than in the narrower definition adopted by practitioners of a particular approach in family therapy, based on the developments in the Milan school of family systemic psychotherapy (e.g., Campbell, 1999).

Clinical practice

This shift to relational thinking has given rise to two powerful developments within the clinical professional field: (a) practice as a qualified family therapist; (b) and/or systemic practice while qualified in another mental health discipline. Both choices are open to mental health professionals who work with individuals, couples, family and extended kin groups, professional teams, agencies, and networks. The systemic paradigm has given rise to a body of well-researched theories and techniques that are helpful to us when offering direct therapy, consultation, training to others and, in our team, working and networking across inter-agency relationships (Boscolo & Bertrando, 1996; Campbell, 1995; Carr, 1997). In this book, we shall consider both professional paths interchangeably when looking at the contribution systemic thinking and practice has made and can make to clinical psychology and the practice of psychotherapy.

Although family therapy had its roots in thinking and working with families, the systemic tradition evolved rapidly as the ideas were seen to have application across a number of different human groupings or systems where the interest lay in thinking about connection and relationships. So, applications with work groups, such as multi-disciplinary teams in major public agencies (Reder, 1986), residential homes (Dimmock & Dungworth, 1985), the educational sector (Dowling & Osborne, 1994), project teams in commerce and industry, management practice (Campbell *et al.*, 1991), inter-agency relationships and working with complex systems (Hardwick, 1991), all led to creative and innovative applications beyond the emotional connections of family relationships. Arguably, this drove the change of description from family therapy to systemic psychotherapy and systemic practice to reflect the diversity, evolution, and range of application of these ideas. In this book, we shall not attempt to try and capture the full flavour of the field as it is today, but rather to concentrate on those developments, ideas, and practices that will be most helpful to applied psychologists, psychotherapists, and mental health practitioners in their day to day practice.

Enduring ideas in systemic family therapy: a conceptual map of the evolution of ideas

Psychology, including clinical psychology, has arguably been fundamentally concerned with the individual and intra-psychic states. This has included the study of cognitive as well as emotional states. Underlying this has been the view that people can be regarded in terms of a relatively stable self, for example, a personality composed of enduring behavioural, cognitive and emotional characteristics. In contrast, one of the most enduring ideas of Systemic Theory is that individual experience, including problems and pathology, is fundamentally interpersonal rather than individual. Philosophically we might question how it is possible to both have individual experience and to say it is not personal and individual but interpersonal. We might suggest a partial answer to this by pointing to the young infant without language who appears to be inextricably connected to, and synchronized to his mother's behaviours and states (Schaffer, 1977; Stern, 1985). Rather than being an immutable fundamental we might argue that the notion of an individual identity and self is learned or socially constructed (Berger & Luckman, 1973; Gergen, 1985). To quote one of our colleagues, babies are born systemic. Arguably, even in our most private moments, for example, when engaged in writing, thoughts ricochet from thinking about the content of what we are trying to write to the potential reactions of the reader.

Though the enduring paradigm shift offered by systemic theory has been the move from an intra- to an interpersonal view of problems and difficulties, there has also been a rich variety of developments and elaborations of this paradigm. These evolutions in many ways parallel some of the changes that have also occurred in mainstream psychology. We want briefly to offer a conceptual map of the developments of family therapy and draw out some of these parallels before we go on to outline some of the core ideas. As a caution we quote the famous phrase much used in family therapy that the map is not the territory (Korzybski, 1942). By this we mean that we are not making a claim that this map objectively represents the reality of the developments but rather that it may capture some of the essence of the changes that have occurred.

Broadly, we suggest that systemic family therapy has progressed through three phases.

Phase 1: systems theory and functional analysis

In many ways the first phase of family therapy can be seen as sharing some perspectives with theory and practice in other types of clinical work. The guiding metaphor of a family as a system, though representing some fundamental changes in thinking of problems as interpersonal versus intra-personal, nevertheless can be seen as containing some of the dominant contemporary ideas. For example, a central idea was that a symptom displayed by one member of a family was serving a "function", such as a family which might otherwise disintegrate into separations or divorce, so that it is able to assist and care for the person. This idea is shared by behavioural approaches and psychodynamic therapies. In addition, families were conceptualized in terms of behavioural sequences and patterns and in emphasizing the function of a symptom in maintaining the stability of a family system. Significantly, therapy involved a belief that family systems could be accurately described in terms of such patterns and structures and the therapist, as an expert, could initiate changes largely outside the family's awareness. There were differences, too, in that systemic approaches emphasized communication, not just behaviour. In fact, behaviours were seen as a form of communication or exchange of information in families. However, family members' unconscious responses to each other's communications were given considerable emphasis, in contrast to their more explicit understandings of their own and each other's actions.

Types of therapy

- Structural.
- Strategic.
- Brief Therapy.

Focus

- Function of symptoms in the family.

Core concepts

- Circular versus linear causality.
- Dysfunctional patterns and structures.
- Circularities (patterns of behaviour).
- Family structures.
- Power, inequalities and confusions.
- Homeostasis.
- Family rules.
- Communication.

Key therapeutic approaches

- Therapeutic tasks.
- Altering patterns.
- Disrupting circularities.
- Reframing.
- Altering structures.
- Unbalancing.
- Enactment.

Phase 2: constructivism

This represented a move, again in many ways consistent with changes outside systemic family therapy. For example, psychology saw a shift, that came to be known as the cognitive revolution, to a focus on cognition, meaning, and personal beliefs as opposed to the dominance of a behavioural approach. The notion of an observable, objectively known family was questioned in favour of a view of the therapist as only being able, like the family members themselves, to form personal, subjective views. A core metaphor in this phase of family therapy came to be of the person in a kind of "personal biosphere". This suggested that each person essentially held a unique and personal view of the world. In turn, each family member was seen as unique and possessing a unique view of their family, expectations of each other, and so on. Therapeutically, this phase significantly entailed a move away from the therapist as expert to a more collaborative position. The therapist recognized that he or she might never really understand how members of a family saw things, partly due to the complexity of this task but, most importantly, also because this understanding would itself be coloured by his or her own assumptions and prejudices.

Types of therapy

- Milan.
- Family Construct Psychology.
- Brief Therapy/Solution-focused therapy.

Focus

- Patterns of beliefs in families.
- Levels of meanings.
- Communication.
- Observing systems.
- Hypothesizing.

Core concepts

- Punctuation.
- Reality as subjective.
- Inter-locking beliefs.
- Auto-poiesis.
- Communication.

Key therapeutic approaches

- Reframing.
- Re-storying.
- Co-construction of shared stories.
- Circular questioning.
- Positive connotation.

Phase 3: social constructionism

Again reflecting changes in sociology and psychology, especially social psychology, there was a move towards seeing families and individuals as inextricably linked to the wider cultural contexts, especially through our participation in language. This included a growing recognition of how normative assumptions about family life are embedded in the language of any given culture. It is argued that language contains a legacy of ideas, for example, assumptions relating to gender, race, and class. In some ways this third phase brought back into focus notions of commonality (as in the first phase) of family experience versus the individuality emphasized by the second phase. However, now these were seen to be shaped by the immersion of the family in the wider socio-political and socio-linguistic realities rather than being predominantly internally produced.

Types of therapy

- Feminist.
- Narrative.
- Post-Milan.

Focus

- Role of language in shaping experience and actions.

Core concepts

- Discourses.
- Narratives.
- Conversation.
- Reflection.
- Power (socially constructed).

Key therapeutic approaches

- Re-storying.
- Reflecting processes (teams).
- Externalizing problems.
- Interviewing the internalized other.
- Writing.

It is possible to see in this map close parallels with developments in psychology. The dominance of behavioural models in both clinical and academic psychology gave way in the 1970s to the "cognitive revolution". In many ways the development of cognitive psychology in academic psychology was mirrored in clinical psychology by the ascent of cognitive therapeutic approaches, not least cognitive behavioural therapy (CBT) (Beck, 1967). Although still arguably dominant, these in turn have been followed by models and practice influenced by the ascent of social constructionism and ideas about mindfulness. Significantly, we have seen the contribution of a critical position inspired by feminist thinking and more broadly by socio-linguistic approaches, such as Foucault's analysis of the interconnected role of language and power. Of course, these developments have not been discrete but can be seen as gaining ascendancy and influence over particular periods. For example, social constructionist ideas complement the earlier critiques of psychiatry in the anti-psychiatry movement that questioned the relevance and practices of biomedical models and their emphasis on diagnosis and attendant medical interventions.

We will argue in this volume that one of the important contributions to clinical practice is the skill of critical integration of models. Although to a lesser extent than in, for example, clinical psychology, there have also been attempts within the field of family therapy to develop integrated approaches. Importantly, this has included an attempt to reintroduce the person and personal experience as a central feature of systemic family therapy. So, as in clinical psychology, for example, family therapy has moved (first phase) from a focus on pattern and behaviour with little attention given to internal experiences to a primary concern with meaning, internal experience, and subjectivity (second phase). This also contained a shift in emphasis from positivist and nomothetic approaches that were interested in the search for commonalities and general laws to an emphasis on individuality and uniqueness. However, within clinical psychology, CBT, for example, perhaps represented a hybrid that maintained a commitment to a search for general explanations for types of depressive cognitions. In the third phase intra-psychic experience is still central, both in clinical psychology and family therapy, but there is also a recognition of commonalities of experience shaped by the language in any given culture. In return there is recognition of issues of power and inequality and their implications for regimes of practice.

More recently, practitioners have welcomed attempts to look at integrative ways of working which span different models of psychotherapy: Dallos (1991)—personal construct therapy and systemic psychotherapy; Vetere and Henley (2001)—group analytic psychotherapy and systemic psychotherapy; Wachtel and Wachtel —(1986) behaviour therapy and psychodynamic psychotherapy, and psychodynamic and systemic; Byng-Hall (1995)—systemic and attachment theory, and so on. In addition, there has been some rapprochement between models that have in the past defined different territories of thinking and practice, such as the fields of psychoanalysis and systemic psychotherapy (Larner, 2000). Arguably, a systemic framework is ideally suited to help both integrative projects and attempts at rapprochement, based as it is in general system theory (von Bertalanffy, 1968) with its potential to work as meta-theory. As a meta-theory, general system theory provides helpful guidelines and a language within which to make links between different theoretical models (Vetere & Gale, 1987).

The development of critical psychology (Fox & Prilleltensky, 1997) and the post-modern critiques of psychotherapeutic practice provide a stimulating forum within which to review the more recent contributions of systemic thinking and practice (Hayward, 1996; Pilgrim, 2000; Pocock, 1996). Contributions from those practitioners who write about their interest in working with issues of difference, such as cultural differences, gender differences, issues of disability, sexuality, age, and religion, have offered a number of critical perspectives on many "taken for granted" assumptions in all psychotherapy practices (Dallos & Dallos, 1997). In particular, we think the critiques of power relations in society, at all levels of relationship, have been the most demanding and challenging of all our practices (Burck & Speed, 1995). Thus, one of our tasks in this book is to evaluate how well we think the family and systemic psychotherapies have fared under this intense scrutiny.

Observing families

As in several social science fields, many of the fundamental ideas are developed early. Often what seems to follow are elaborations and critiques rather than substantial shifts. Arguably, this is nowhere more true than in systemic family therapy. One of the fundamental ideas was to emphasize the importance of patterns in behaviour, patterns over time, and the rules for behaviour and beliefs that might be said to underpin those patterns. The crux of a systemic analysis lies in the connections postulated between pattern, behaviour, and beliefs at a relational level of description and explanation. As in the development of behaviourism the fundamental starting point for family therapy was the observation of behaviour. The early ideas arose from research into communicational processes in families and, importantly, this observational research was significantly facilitated by the rapidly increasing availability of visual recording methods, especially videotape.

Later in this section, and in Chapter Two, we shall outline some core systemic techniques that provide the means to explore the veracity of systemic thinking in interaction with family members.

Pattern in relationships

Systemic theory offered an important conceptual shift in our understanding of human behaviour and experience. This has been described as a shift from linear to circular causation. Rather than offering explanations which typically featured cause and effect sequences, such as:

Linear:

John is depressed because he lost his job.

Or

➡ John's personality makes him prone to depression.

circular explanations emphasize recursive connections between events and experiences, such as:

Circular:

In reaction to John losing his job his friends tried to help him and cheer him up, which made him feel incompetent, leading him to feel more depressed and in turn soliciting more sympathy ... leading him to become angry and withdrawn ... eventually avoidance by his friends ... and more depressed.

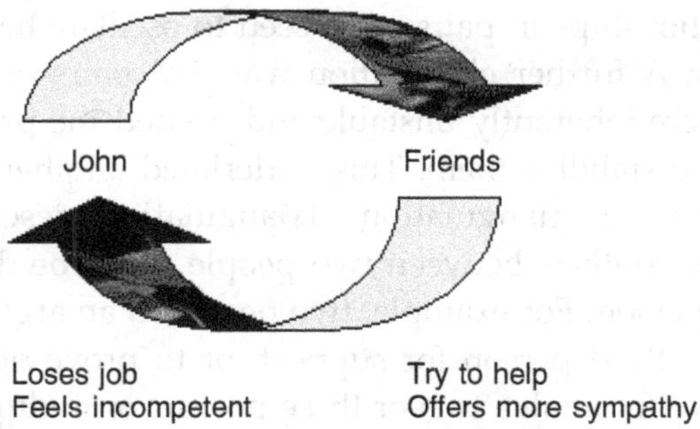

The above examples are simplifications but offer the idea of interconnection and, importantly, the connected idea that we are continually involved in patterns of interactional processes. (See also Watzlawick *et al.*'s (1974) concept of punctuation.)

Escalation and feedback

In this example we can see some of the core ideas of a systemic perspective—escalation and feedback. The two sets of actions are interconnected so that John and his friends mutually influence each others' actions and reactions in such a way that the situation escalates. More specifically, two patterns of escalation have been observed:

1. Complementarity. These are patterns where participants act in different but matched ways. An example might be where one person is accusative and the other apologetic or defensive, or where one initiates and the other follows. Arguably, abusive relationships often have this form, where one is dominant and the other submissive. The extent to which a "victim" can be said to contribute to this abusive pattern has been a contentious issue (Goldner *et al.*, 1990; Williams & Watson, 1988).
2. Symmetrical. These have a sense of competition, in which each participant acts in a similar way. For example, in an escalating argument each person shouts, gestures, and threatens with increasing intensity. Another example, might be where two people mutually complain of how ill they are, or two people compete over telling the funniest joke, or giving the best compliment.

Relationships in pairs were seen to oscillate between those two patterns. A further observation was that pairs or dyadic relationships were inherently unstable and needed the presence of a third person to stabilize them. This underlined another influential early idea, that of triangulation. Triangulation described a process whereby conflicts between two people could be detoured through a third person. For example, two people in an argument may try to pull in a third person for support, or to prove one of them right. Patterns can involve two or three people, or multiple relationships.

In a search to describe and explain such observations of various relationships, ideas from systems theory were incorporated. Systems theory had been developed in the fields of biology and control engineering to explain both patterns of escalation and also balance (homeostasis). A biological example is the maintenance of heart rate. Although this may increase or decrease according to activity, it is maintained through various mechanisms within safe limits, protecting the heart and the body from serious damage.

Homeostasis

One of the seminal early ideas was that in addition to escalating patterns, which were termed *open systems*, family relationships could be seen as closed or stable systems. Significantly, Jackson (1957) argued that in a perverse way a family could become organized so that the interactions served "as if" to maintain a problem. For example, problems displayed by a young child could function to distract the parents from their own escalating conflicts and distress and unite them in their mutual concern for the child. If such a solution to a problem persisted over time it could lead to the child's problem becoming chronic. Importantly, this cast a new light on the common clinical phenomenon of resistance. Rather than viewing this as an internal, intra-psychic state, it could now be seen in terms of the inertia of the system. For example, the cessation of the child's symptoms might imply a threat (perhaps experienced unconsciously) that the couple might have to confront their own problems. There might also be a concomitant fear in the child that her parents' relationship might disintegrate. Interestingly, these early systemic ideas made connections with psychodynamic ideas; for example, the idea of the family myth which distorted reality into the belief that the child's symptoms were the cause rather than the consequence of the family's problems. Jackson went on to propose that families in which symptoms were contained could be described as homeostatic systems. He suggested that this entailed the family operating and obeying a set of rules stating that things must stay the same. At times these early ideas were employed in a rather mechanistic manner, but it is important to note that Jackson made clear that he regarded the concept of rules as *propositional*—as a more or less useful way of thinking about families rather than rules as having an objective status.

Triangles and escalation

As our examples above suggest, an important observation was that the fundamental unit of analysis was not the person, or pairs of people, but threesomes or triads. Interestingly, Minuchin (1974) draws on the notion that the basic human group is three, not two. By this he means that whenever two people get together they are influenced by a third, who may be absent geographically, or absent through death. Thus, in understanding relationships, Minuchin would use the relational triangle as a building block on which to understand the interlocking relational triangles in their patterned ways. Watzlawick *et al.* (1967, 1974) suggested that interactions in pairs were inevitably prone to *escalation* and needed to be stabilized by a third party (Figure 1).

Although having an intuitive appeal, the concept of patterns in families also raises many questions. For example, what constitutes a pattern? According to Bateson (1980), pattern can be thought of as sequences of connectedness within and between people that have behavioural, emotional, and cognitive aspects; or pattern in relationships between people, events, beliefs, and behaviours. Looking for patterns can be seen as the way we make sense of our world, "We think with the aid of pattern" (Bateson, 1980).

As therapists, exploring patterns with family members inevitably means selecting certain sequences above others as we distinguish figure from ground. In the early stages of the development of family therapy, therapists observed interactional patterns in families, identified those that seemed to be maintaining a problem and intervened to alter them. The more rigidly patterned

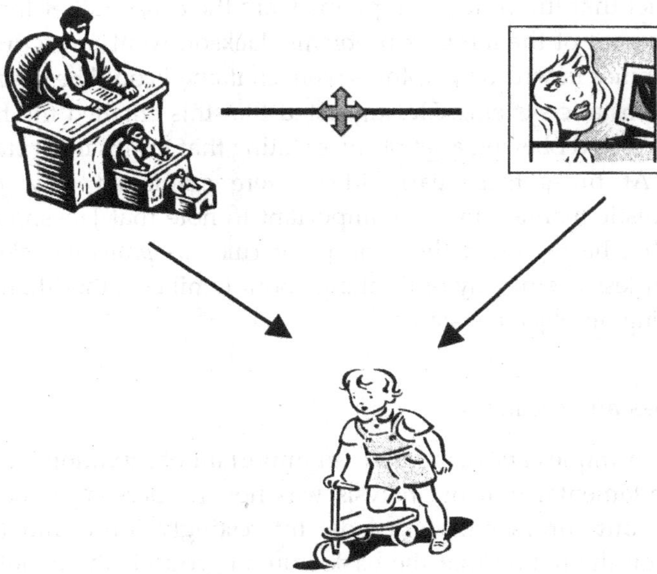

Figure 1. The function of a third party in stabilizing conflicting interactions between pairs.

the family's interactions, the less adaptable the family members were considered to be, and at greater risk of interpersonal difficulty in the face of external demands for change.

In the second phase of family therapy, there was a vigorous reappraisal of the concept of pattern. We were reminded that some of us had slipped into making assumptions that patterns really existed in an identifiable way. Ideas from constructivist psychology reminded us that patterns do not exist "out there" as such, but more in the inferences we form and share with others. This led to the idea of the therapist observer as part of the system and reminds us that the patterns we observe are only one of many possible sequences we could identify (Hoffman, 1993). The way we construe those patterns will affect our formulations, our discussions, our interventions and the family members' responses in an iterative process over the course of the therapy. A therapist observer who joins a system with an emotionally significant shared history, such as a family, will inevitably notice patterns that those engaged in daily interactions with each other are less likely to notice. By choosing to identify and intervene in problematic patterns, family therapists can avoid blaming individuals, invite their clients to be curious about their loyalty to particular patterns, and consider what alternatives they might have. This might include speculating about what would happen if one of the participants in the interaction suddenly changed their behaviour.

Members of family groups and other systems often act *as if* they are organized by rules which govern the parameters of behaviour (Jackson, 1957), such as rules about what behaviours and interactions are permissible. These rules might be overt, such as rules for children's behaviour, or covert, such as a rule that conflict can only be expressed indirectly. Family members may ask for professional help when rules have become rigid and constraining, such as at times of life-cycle or other transitions, for example, children in stepfamilies may retain loyalties to rules in the previous family when the new family is trying to develop new rules (Gorell Barnes *et al.*, 1998). Thus, for systemic thinkers, how a behavioural pattern is given meaning depends on the context (see Reflexive note 2).

Beliefs and punctuation

Initially, family systems theory adopted a behavioural/biological orientation, but at the same time it emphasized that meanings and beliefs held by family members played a crucial role in regulating their actions and feelings. So, if we accept the notion that some interpersonal behaviour in families can be described *as if* it is rule governed (Goffman, 1971; Harre & Secord, 1972), we need in addition to explore the beliefs that might be said to underpin and support such rules, particularly if family members wish to challenge and modify them. Beliefs can be described as the premises that we use to make sense of our world and which act as invisible guidelines in families for how to behave (Dallos, 1991; Procter, 1981; Reiss, 1980).

Beliefs that play a central part in organizing what behaviours are possible in daily living may have evolved over generations and will reflect such things as gender and cultural beliefs as well as idiosyncratic family beliefs, for example, that education is wasted on women because they get married and have children, or that grandparents can do a better job of caring for children, or that first-born sons are expected to take responsibility. Most centrally in our work with families, we find that many are struggling with ideas that their problems are due to some form of biological or organic deficit, when there appears to be no supportive evidence for this belief. Typically, these ideas might include notions that one member has a "mental illness" or has inherited a particular (and undesirable?) personality trait. Frequently, we hear adolescent boys described as moody and aggressive, and just like their fathers, who may have been in trouble with the law most of their lives. In part, these beliefs could be seen as internalizations of popular discourses about problems. For example, the prominence currently given to genetics research may support a belief that all problems will be traceable to medical/organic factors.

In our everyday use of language, we have few words that help us to describe relationships or our lived experience within a relationship, that do not reflect individual characteristics and traits. For example, we talk of "happy marriages" and "unhappy marriages", or "poor relationships", "volatile/exciting" or "abusive" relationships. However, there are relatively few concepts that enable us to describe the patterns or dynamics of relationships. As we saw above, one example of relationship descriptions is the notion of escalation in terms of symmetrical patterns, or complementary patterns (Watzlawick *et al.*, 1967, Weakland *et al.*, 1974). We should note that these patterns may also reflect positions of equity and power-sharing in relationships, namely reciprocal relationships. This language allows us to speak of symmetrical relationships, where two persons actively strive in competition, say, to have the last word, or to exchange the best compliment, whereas a complementary relationship describes a power imbalance where one of the participants holds the balance of power in decision making and in defining the nature of the relationship. Some complementary relationships are socially sanctioned, such as employer–employee or parent–child, with legal frameworks to try and prevent abuses of power. Reciprocal relationships are thought to capture equity in relationships, where at times one person might have more power than the other, but overall there is a balance of power. Another example is found in the work of Minuchin (1974). He described relationships in terms of a continuum of emotional closeness and emotional distance. Minuchin thought that relationships could be described to move along the continuum according to a number of factors, such as respective roles, age, gender, cultural demands, and so on. For example, a baby and primary care-taker might be described within an emotionally very close relationship that, with the passage of time, maturational changes and societal demands, becomes less emotionally intense as the child develops other relationships, including intimate relationships in adolescence and adulthood.

To understand patterns of relationships between families and professionals, it is useful to explore families', professionals' and agency-wide beliefs about receiving help from outsiders and offering help to families, while drawing on Bateson's (1972) language for describing power relations. We may find a complementary fit between sets of beliefs, where families have evolved a pattern of family life that includes depending on Social Services for support and where social workers think their task is to support families. In this instance, the fit may be too good, in that it is difficult for the family members and the social workers to disengage. Or we may find a symmetrical pattern in relationships between family members and Social Services where the family resists Social Services' intervention, leading to an escalation of anxiety and perceived lack of cooperation, often culminating in care proceedings.

Family therapists and systemic practitioners have a long tradition of being interested in both content and process, and trying to hold the tension between both sources of information in communication. In conducting a systemic interview, for example, family therapists may be less concerned with *content* i.e. the individual accounts given by different family members than with *process* i.e. the ways in which these different accounts connect to the patterns of relationship observed, or the ways in which these accounts are told and retold in interaction. Thus the content of an argument between family members, say about a difference of opinion, may sometimes be seen as less important than the *ways* in which family members seem to habitually conduct their differences. Such a view of process invites us to pay attention to non-verbal behaviour, and allows room for us to consider the complexities of human behaviour. Where content would take precedence over process might be when working with issues of abuse and violence between family members. We shall return to these issues, when we discuss issues of power in relationships and in particular when we consider the case of working with violent behaviour.

Change

As we have seen, a fundamental idea from systems theory was the suggestion by Don Jackson (1957) that relationships which contained "pathology" could be seen to function as closed systems. These operated so that any change in the symptomatic member would be met by actions in the others that would have the sum effect of reducing, rather than encouraging, change. Despite family members expressing a desire to change, it was argued that in some sense the symptom had been incorporated into the relationship dynamics, and the habitual behaviour in relation to the symptoms served to maintain, rather than change, the problems.

However, systemic thinking has developed to suggest that change can take place at a number of inter-related levels:

- Behavioural patterns—this was the initial emphasis on structure and processes in families.
- Belief systems—the beliefs, explanations, and understanding are seen to underlie family processes and shifts in these can lead to profound changes.
- Emotional patterns—include the emotional atmosphere in a family, the level of emotional arousal and volatility, and can also include the nature of the emotional attachments.
- Relationship with wider contexts—families live within wider cultural and political contexts with expectations about what is seen as acceptable and non-acceptable behaviour. Change in these systems may also need to occur if families are not simply being coerced into accepting potentially oppressive ideals.

Change can be seen to involve an interplay of all these domains of change. So, for example, a family may need to experience a level of emotional calm before they start to alter their beliefs and behaviours. This may also help them to reflect on the wider ideas that shape their lives together and in some cases to take action to resist, for example, racist or sexist assumptions. Most importantly, change is not simply objective but is also a subjective process.

Different people observing a family may see different types of change occurring, or not, as the case may be. A therapist needs to be cautious in making assumptions about what kind of change has occurred or should occur. Returning to our three-phase map for a moment, we can summarize some of the views regarding change:

- First phase—change and *stuckness* are seen predominantly in terms of the dynamics within the family—structures, processes, beliefs, and attachments. One aspect of this can be a tendency to view families negatively and engage in blaming—they are "resistant", "poorly motivated", "too damaged", and so on.
- Second phase—change and "stuckness" can be considered more in terms of the family–therapist system. "Stuckness" is seen in terms of interactions between the therapist and family, failed interventions, failure of the therapeutic alliance. In addition, change is seen essentially to involve a shift in beliefs and understandings.
- Third phase—change and "stuckness" are seen predominantly in terms of societal processes, for example, gender and racial inequalities, contradictions inherent in the culture which are not simply "fixable" but require a process of exposure and resistance. The therapist is seen as working with the family to expose contradictory and oppressive beliefs and discourses which have been internalized by the family and therapy team and shape common "stuck" dynamics. Change is seen to happen partly through liberation—therapy as partly a "political" process.

A further summary is offered by Fraser (1995), who has developed some useful ideas in relation to a process view of change that underpin some problem-solving and solution-focused approaches to systemic practice. They can be summarized as follows:

(a) process is a patterned flow of concepts and related actions seen in interaction;
(b) change is a continual process, with both process and evolution seen as primary;
(c) change is often quite rapid;
(d) "structures" and "systems" are thought to be products of describers, and thus depend on and include the observer; just as

meaning is thought to be variable and a product of describers and their emergent interaction;

(e) underlying pathology is not assumed;
(f) problems are escalating positive feedback cycles of concept and action around attempts to assimilate or accommodate some variation; thus, there are many starting points and paths to the development of problems;
(g) there are multiple useful interaction patterns; thus, there are many useful resolutions to problems; and
(h) small changes in concept and action often lead to more positive "ripples" via positive feedback processes.

This emphasis on process means exploring presenting difficulties not as fixed categories, such as depression or low self-esteem, but as contextualized by relationships and beliefs at individual, family, and cultural levels of explanation. For example, questions could be asked such as: "How do you treat your partner differently when you think he or she is depressed?", or, "Who in the family has high self-esteem?" Family therapy therefore aims to make new connections between beliefs, behaviour, and relationships. We shall discuss systemic hypothesizing and the use of circular questions later in the book.

Communication

Watzlawick *et al.*, (1974) put forward the idea that all behaviour is communication, that it is impossible to "not communicate". Communication is thought to occur on at least two levels. By thinking about both content and process, we can also juxtapose the verbal or report level of the message with the command or relationship level of the message, that is, the implicit and explicit rules about how the message is to be construed and who sets those rules. Thus, it could be said that the relationship level of the message acts as the context for the report level of the message. These levels are thought not to be the same, and if they are treated as if they are the same, then the effect is confusing or paradoxical, for example, "all statements in this book are false". The nature of our interpersonal relationships is thought to influence how we might make sense of sequences of communication. Punctuation is a term used to denote how we come to understand and give meaning to what we experience. Such an approach suggests that over time punctuation becomes a pattern. Once we are very familiar with a pattern it becomes "natural" for us to think and understand in particular ways.

This long-standing interest in process/content distinctions is seen in systemic ideas of communication. The work of Watzlawick and colleagues (1974) described above drew our attention to the report and command characteristics of a message. In everyday interaction, we are often faced with situations where someone says something to us that they seem to contradict non-verbally, for example, telling us they are not angry through clenched teeth. These apparent report/command contradictions in communicative behaviour are the stuff of our therapeutic conversations. It has been suggested that when we cannot comment directly on the apparent contradiction in the communication, (for example, the statement "all statements in this book are false"), say, because we do not hold power in the relationship, and are overly dependent on the relationship for our welfare and well-being, that we find ourselves in a double-bind (Bateson *et al.*, 1956). Double-binding communications are thought to impair emotional development and a sense of a coherent self when they dominate key interactions for children on psychologically significant topics. In relationships characterized by reciprocity, we pay more attention to content, the "what" of what we are saying, rather than the command aspects of the message, which are more to do with the definition of the relationship in terms of power. In our clinical practice, double-binding communication can be troubling, for example, when a client repeatedly telephones to say he does not want an appointment, or when family members want the symptom changed but not the family.

Patterns over time

An influential model of change and development was proposed in the concept of the family life-cycle. This emphasized how development and change in families followed common patterns that were shaped by the shifting patterns of internal and external demands in any society. Family members may at times be faced with massive demands for change and adaptation. This may be a result of changes in family composition—the birth of a child, marital separation, death, or remarriage: or perhaps be due to changes of autonomy within the family—children becoming adults, a woman returning to external employment after child rearing, or retirement. It was argued that the emergence of problems was frequently associated with these life-cycle transitions and their inherent demands and stresses. However, less was said about the possible positive effect of external inputs, for example, the arrival of a baby possibly uniting a couple, or a bereavement drawing family members closer together. Without an analysis of the meanings such events held for family members, accounts of change tended to be merely descriptive. A key issue for any family was how to maintain some form of identity and structure while at the same time needing to continually evolve, adapt, change, and respond to external stimuli. There may also be community demands such as local social upheavals and major cultural changes.

Duvall (1957) extended the idea of the individual life-cycle model to the idea of a family life-cycle. The implications of this model for the practice of family therapy were first set out by Haley (1973) in his book describing the therapeutic techniques of Milton Erickson (see Second phase, p. 11). Haley describes how Milton Erickson had noted that problems were often associated with critical periods of change and transition in families. For example, psychotic experiences in late adolescence were seen to be related to difficulties for the family over the departure of the young person about to leave and set up his or her own home. Haley described the following stages as critical, transitional stages for families: birth of a child; leaving home; independent living; marriage; retirement.

Family life-cycle models

In this section we shall introduce the concepts of (a) the family life-cycle; (b) repetitive generational patterns of behaviour; and (c) family "scripts".

Family life-cycle models emphasize the evolution of family relationships over time. A life-span analysis is advocated by some when working with individuals (Erickson, 1968). The individual life-cycle occurs for many of us within the extended family life-cycle, considered to be one of the primary contexts of human social, emotional and cognitive development (Carter & McGoldrick, 1989).

According to Carter and McGoldrick, the processes for family members to negotiate are the expansion, contraction, and realignment of the relationship systems to support the entry, exit, and development of family members in an adaptive way. They provide a view of the life-cycle in terms of inter-generational connectedness in the family. Separately domiciled families are seen by Carter and McGoldrick as emotional subsystems, reacting to past, present and future relationships within the larger three–four generational extended family system. They recognize, both theoretically and therapeutically, connectedness in life—within any type of family structure—with those who went before and those who follow.

Processes of change are required of family members at each possible transition in the family life-cycle, for example, birth or adoption of a child, marriage or cohabitation, leaving home as a young adult, leaving through separation and divorce, death of a family member, retirement, and so on. Change for an individual is thought to make changes necessary in some relationships and to provide the opportunity for change in others for example, the transition into adolescence can upset prevailing stability and require significant adjustments in family relationships. This approach views psychological distress and symptoms in the context of the evolution of family relationships. The prime therapeutic task is seen as enabling the family to re-establish developmental momentum. Further problems may be caused when family systems are making changes in the structure and function of their relationships in advance of recognition of those changes at social systems levels.

Family life-cycle thinking does not intend that a judgemental view of a normal/abnormal continuum of changes throughout the family life-cycle should be taken. Rather, it is important to note similarities and differences for the rich diversity of family forms, for example, stepfamilies, lone parent families, extended kin groups, adopting families, religious and ethnic differences, and so on. Family life-cycle thinking can be seen as a starting point for looking at culturally specific tasks and functions for each family member at different family life-cycle stages, however defined, and the demands of these transitions as family members develop in relation to one another.

Byng-Hall (2000) has written about the helpfulness of tracing developmental pathways with couples and parents in therapy. His questioning is designed to elucidate the cultural template (Nock, 2000) for family life held by those in the therapy, thus comparing the older cultural expectations of the steps through which a family should pass with the steps that the couple or family group have taken thus far. He explores the experiences they might have missed, or have altered, and the consequences for family members. He might further ask the couple what phases in their relationship they think they have been through, how they have managed them, and whether they have needed to alter and adapt their expectations and behaviours as a result. Thus, Byng-Hall combines the framework of life-cycle stages and developmental pathways with an enquiring approach that attempts to map whether the ideas hold validity for the couple in their understanding of their relationships and the emotional contexts within which they develop.

Some core ideas in the life-cycle model

1. The stages in the family life-cycle are somewhat arbitrary and recent; for example, adolescence is considered by some historians to be a nineteenth-century invention (Aries, 1962); young adulthood as an independent phase a twentieth-century invention (Stainton-Rogers & Stainton-Rogers, 1992); women as independent persons a late twentieth-century phenomenon (Radcliffe Richards, 1980). In addition, "launching children and moving on" is the newest and longest phase, affected by changing economic circumstances and employment opportunities; and more women are living through the older age phase. Factors such as longer life expectancy, divorce and remarriage rates and the changing role of women, among others, contribute to these developments. Family members may well find there are few available models of the passages they are going through, as well as a lack of some transitional rituals and markers. Nock (2000) suggests that family members today do not have many templates for family life compared with more traditionally structured families of a few generations ago. The rise of contraceptive practice and the choices that couples make about whether or when to have children put responsibility firmly within the couple relationship where the consequences of such choices are not clearly

defined. This freedom to decide, according to Nock, has interesting consequences. He sees the rise in popularity of couples and family work to be largely in response to the deconstruction of cultural templates.

If we consider that three–four generations may be accommodating to life-cycle transitions simultaneously (for example, older age, children leaving home, young adulthood, "arriving" in the system), we can see that different cohorts born and living through different periods may differ in fertility, mortality, migration patterns, education, acceptable gender roles, economic resources, moral values, and so on. Therapists can often overlook the life-shaping impact of one generation on another; for example, the impact of changes in the grandparent generation, such as increasing physical frailty, on the next generation (household) group who might be the group in therapy. Although the structure, stages, and form of the household group are subject to social and demographic changes, the relationship patterns and family themes continue to sound familiar.

2. Some critics have argued that any stage theory of human development contains within it the potential for misuse. For example, the pitfalls of rigid application of life-cycle theories include the tendency to see any deviation from "normal" as pathological; conversely, the overemphasis of the uniqueness of each generation can promote historical discontinuity with little relationship acknowledged between the generations. Life-cycle models have been adapted in response to criticisms that they describe Western, wealthy, nuclear families, and have not properly considered the importance of difference, both economically and culturally (McGoldrick *et al.*, 1991).

3. Each posited family life-cycle stage presents family members with different functions, tasks, and role complexes in relation to one another. During the stages between the transitional points in the evolution of a family there may appear habitual patterns of interaction that are more likely to be predictable and repetitive. Such processes are likely to be consistent with belief systems and current definitions of relationships. Negative feedback processes are likely to operate, i.e., those that ensure stability within the system.

4. Family members are required to negotiate transitions between the stages. Transitions can be characterized by triggers, timing and the magnitude of change (such as first and second order changes). Triggers are "the comings and goings of family members", the formation of new relationships, and other developments within the system. Family life-cycle theories recognize that exits from the system (examples: death, leaving home, migration, emotional cut-off) give rise to experiences of loss as well as necessitating the reorganization and redefinition of relationships; similarly, entrances (examples: birth, coupling, and marriage) require the realignment of existing relationships. These processes are interactive; for example, the formation of one relationship may depend on the collapse of another, or leaving may be prompted by an arrival.

The timing of transitions can be both expected (biological and social maturation in children, socially prescribed changes in roles, family scripts, cultural and religious rituals to mark transitions) and unexpected (untimely life events). Positive feedback processes are likely to operate during transitional periods, whereby feedback on the effects of the changes may lead to further changes. The successful negotiation of transitions requires a balance between the processes of stability and change; family members experience varying degrees of loyalty to the past and trepidation/excitement about the future.

Family stress/stressors are believed to be greatest at the time of transition; for example, vertical and horizontal stressors. Vertical stressors are the patterns of relating and functioning transmitted down the generations of a family primarily through the mechanism of emotional triangulation, such as family attitudes, myths, taboos, expectations, and labels. Horizontal stressors are those that arise within and outside the family; for example, predictable developmental stresses and unpredictable life events; and the social, physical and political context in which the life-cycle is enacted. The interaction between vertical and horizontal stressors can determine how well transitions are managed by family members. Given stresses that exceed resources, any family could be seen to have difficulty managing transitions.

5. The systemic view of symptoms and psychological distress that emerges around the time of a transition is that they can serve the

function of preventing change in the family. Limited conflict resolution skills within a family group can make it harder to negotiate a transitional period. The solutions developed for one set of tasks at one stage may become obsolete at another stage; for example, parenting a 15-year-old as though they were much younger. Parents can often "lose" their time/historical perspective during transitional crises, forgetting their own earlier experiences or those of their parents and carers. Drawing on earlier experiences of negotiating crises and transitions can be a helpful resource in the present.

6. The tasks of therapy are to find ways of helping families re-establish developmental momentum. The genogram is used as an assessment and therapeutic tool (Lieberman, 1979; McGoldrick & Gerson, 1989). Therapists recognize the importance of rituals, both religious and secular, designed by families in every culture to ease the passage of members from one status or role to the next.

Genograms are used to highlight patterns and themes that have been occurring in families across the generations and may be influencing present interactions. It was Murray Bowen (see Kerr & Bowen, 1988) who first wrote of the importance of tracking family patterns through their life-cycle over several generations, focusing primarily on nodal events and transition points in family development when seeking to understand family dilemmas and difficulties in the present. Interestingly, Bowen also emphasized, primarily as a result of his continuing interest in psychodynamic models, the interpersonal worlds of family members. In particular, he emphasizes the need for a child to differentiate him or herself from parents, especially the main carer. Failure to develop a sense of self-identity was seen as potentially leading to an inability to become autonomous and to be able to engage in adult relationships. He went on to develop the metaphor of an undifferentiated ego mass to describe particular emotional dynamics in some families; for example, a young adult who continued to be over-involved with his mother, unsure of his self, of his ability to make sense of the world, and to function in the world. Such parent–child patterns were seen as evolving over generations and potentially leading to severe disorders, such as the diagnosis of schizophrenia.

Family scripts

The concept of "family scripts" draws upon ideas from drama and literature. Goffman (1971) had introduced ideas of personal experience and relationships as being shaped by scripts that could function at conscious or unconscious levels. Similarly, this bears resemblance to the concept of "roles", which came from the work of the symbolic interactionists (Mead, 1934). Their ideas of people acting out a variety of roles—that of father, sister, colleague, lover, neighbour, friend, and so on—in different contexts, continues to have a powerful influence in the social sciences and psychological therapies.

The concept of a family script combines the idea of people in families playing multiple roles as if they were actors in a drama. These dramas are seen as set out for us in culturally shared stories, not least in powerful ones derived from dramas such as the stories of *Hamlet,* Oedipus Rex, *Cinderella,* and "The Prodigal Son". More specifically, families are thought to hand on stories across the generations; for example, refugee families' stories of continually moving and fleeing from danger and adversity, stories of success and achievement, stories of insiders and outsiders, or stories of passion or unrequited love. Such stories are thought to be handed on both explicitly, through teaching and example, and implicitly, through expectations and mores. For example, in RD's family, he experienced a script of marriages ending in acrimonious divorce, and of young children fleeing with their mothers from male brutality. Byng-Hall (1998) has described how we typically hold "replicative" or "corrective" positions regarding these scripts; for example, in wanting to be different and do better, to convert the script in our and the next generation. Alternatively, we may choose to repeat or replicate such scripts, or perhaps find ourselves inadvertently doing so. He further argues that how this happens is in turn shaped not just by conscious choices we are able to make, but by patterns of emotional attachments. For example, experience of divorce and emotional uncertainty as a child may shape a self-fulfilling script through the insecurity and inability to trust in the love of subsequent partners.

One idea put forward to describe some of these changes has been that of the "family ledger" (Boszormenyi-Nagy, 1987). This suggests that family members act as if there is a balance book across the generations. For example, if my experience has been that my parents were too unreliable and volatile, I might try to correct for this in the next generation by being more consistent and stable for my children. In turn, they might feel their upbringing was too stable and unexciting and decide that their children need more fun and excitement and be more "open" with them emotionally. Related to these ideas, Boszormenyi-Nagy also emphasized the idea of "relational ethics". By this he suggested that, as in the patterns across the generations, there is a sense in families of justice, of what is fair and equitable. This has parallels in social psychology with the classical equity theory of relationships, that is, social exchange theory (Homans, 1961). In a sense we are shaped by ideas of "getting back what we put in". Where there is a strong sense of unbalance or unfairness, this can lead to distress and conflicts. These may be particularly likely to emerge at the life-cycle transitions, where roles in relation to each other in families are shifting. For example, children may be feeling that they deserve to be treated like adults and parents may come to feel that children should now "pay their way"—that they should contribute to the family income, and so on. These new relational contexts may require considerable negotiation and renegotiation at these times.

Reflexive notes

1. In order to illustrate the notion of pattern (see pp. 16–21), think of an interactional pattern you have noticed that you cannot change; think of a pattern that you noticed because it changed; and predict a pattern that you know will change in the future, but cannot know what it will be like—for example, a predictable life-cycle event.
2. Another illustration exercise for you is to think of a rule in your family of origin. How did you learn about this rule? How did the rule affect you? Who could challenge it? Who was it designed to protect? Does the rule affect you now? What family beliefs might have underpinned this rule?
3. As therapists and practitioners, we need to be aware of our own beliefs about relationships and change, how these will be challenged or confirmed by client groups, and how this will affect our interventions. We will hold certain beliefs about the process of change in relationships and how best to facilitate such changes. These beliefs may be at odds with those of our colleagues and employing agency. So, how would we know, and what consequences might these differences hold for our thinking and practice? For example, many psychologists and psychotherapists work in contexts where medical/illness models of human behaviour prevail. The systemic practitioner may need to walk a fine line in constructively exploring the validity of assumptions that may ignore or minimize social factors or even the interaction between organic and social factors.
4. In reconsidering scripts, think of your family of origin: What gender scripts were you aware of? How do they help/hinder you now? How would you describe your current life-cycle stage? What impact does this have on your work? How would you describe your own experiences of negotiating life-cycle transitions? What impact does this have on your work?

CHAPTER TWO

Enduring and helpful techniques in systemic thinking and practice

Family therapy has developed action techniques, such as enactment and sculpting, which help make patterns between people visible, and questioning techniques, such as circular questions, which help to evaluate systemic hypotheses.

Systemic hypothesizing

A systemic hypothesis is an attempt to develop the connections between information gained from family members during a family interview. It will often include information about life-cycle transitions and inter-generational patterns; relationship patterns (closeness and distance) and recent changes in those patterns; family beliefs and the relationship to the presenting difficulties; dilemmas around change; and issues of gender and culture. Systemic hypotheses are developed and discarded as new information emerges or is elaborated in subsequent family meetings. Cecchin (1987) has suggested that when practitioners consider themselves stuck in their work with families, it is either because they have fallen in love with one hypothesis or because they are thinking at one level of the system. Under such circumstances, his advice is to challenge ourselves by broadening the contextual frame for our thinking.

The use of circular questions

Before discussing the use of circular questions, we wish to challenge the notion that in a systemic interview every question asked has to be a "good one". In addition, we wish to clarify when we might ask (a) direct questions, and (b) circular questions.

Circular questions can be used to develop systemic hypotheses and to help evaluate them. Thus, in early meetings with family members, after describing the presenting difficulties, we might ask: who was most keen to seek help for these difficulties; what was it that made them decide to ask for help; and why now; what do other family members think of the decision to seek help; if our agency/ service is unable to be helpful, what will they do; if our agency/ service is able to be helpful, what will this enable them to do. By paying attention to the feedback from family members, including non-verbal communication, we can gradually widen the systemic frame within which we question. Discussing such questions with family members present at the meeting, and predicting how absent family members might respond, reveals useful information about family-wide disagreements and differences about the problem, the events that prompted the decision to seek help, and the life-cycle transitional stage that may be unsettling some family members' preferred ways of relating.

Circular questions have been described as interventive (Tomm, 1984a,b), in that by asking questions of family members in terms of differences and patterns, they make apparent the connections between beliefs, behaviours, events, and relationships. Family members are asked, in turn, to comment on the thoughts, behaviour, and relationships of the other members of the family and of other significant persons. To be useful, they should be linked to systemic hypotheses.

Such questioning can have powerful effects. For example, children may have a variety of responses to circular questions, not least confusion, and a sense that they are stupid and do not know the right answer (Stith *et al.*, 1996; Strickland-Clark *et al.*, 2000). It may be helpful to ask direct questions when asking for feedback from children, and then to introduce them to systemic questioning through facilitating their own spoken curiosity about other points of view. It is important therefore, that the therapist thinks about the potential impact that the questions might have and uses them within an overall set of formulations or hypotheses to help direct and shape their potential contribution.

Burnham (1986)* has classified circular questions into six categories of sequential, action, classification, diachronic, hypothetical, and mind-reading questions.

1. *Sequential questions*. These enquire into specific interactive behaviour in specific circumstances (not in terms of feelings or interpretations). They elicit patterns in which individual distress/problems are embedded. "When your daughter says that life isn't worth living, what does your husband do?" and so on . . .
2. *Action questions*. These enquire into differences as indicated by behaviour rather than descriptions of individual characteristics. Enquire what a person does to earn a particular description. "What does your son say or do that makes you think he's pathetic?"
3. *Classification questions*. These allow the ranking of responses by family members to specific behaviour or specific interactions. They open up enquiry by finding out the differential responses (pleasure, anger, etc.) or beliefs (optimism/pessimism, etc.) of all family members towards a transition, a problem, or an attempted solution. "When your wife said she was fed up with being at home and wanted to get a job, which of your three children, in your opinion, showed most enthusiasm towards the idea?"

   "When your sister stays out all night who in the family do you see getting most annoyed?"

   "Who most believes that putting Johnny in care will solve the problems?"

---

*Reprinted with permission from Burnham, J. (1966). *Family Therapy* (pp. 111–115). London: Routledge.

4. *Diachronic questions*. These investigate changes in behaviour that indicate a change in relationships at two different points in time, i.e. before and after a specific event. "Did Joe and Mummy get close to each other before or after your father died?"
5. *Hypothetical questions*. These look into differences of opinion with respect to imagined situations (past/current/future). "If you went to university, which of your parents do you think would miss you the most?"
6. *Mind-reading questions*. These questions examine the quality of communication in a family, showing the extent to which members are aware of each other's thoughts and feelings. "If your mother were still alive today, what do you think her opinion would be about the problems you are having with the children?"

Reframing

> To reframe, then, means to change the conceptual and/or emotional setting or viewpoint in relation to which a situation is experienced and place it in another frame which fits the 'facts" of the same concrete situation equally well or even better and thereby changes its entire meaning. [Watzlawick *et al.*, 1974]

Reframing as a cognitive technique is used extensively by therapists of many persuasions. Systemic practitioners recognize the power of reframing in creating possibilities for change in relationships and in the relationally-based beliefs that may influence behavioural choices. Often family members will have a lineal or blaming view of the difficulties, such as, "If my partner stopped drinking, we would be a happy family", or "If my partner was not depressed we would have a happy marriage". Our way of explaining a problem will often contribute to maintaining the problem because our attempted solutions are based on the same set of defining premises. Additionally, we may be more likely to become defensive about our position when a problem is framed negatively and thus find it harder to motivate ourselves to change.

Family therapists use reframing to redefine problems as interactional, thus "she is a problem" becomes "you are having a problem with her ...". Some difficulties can be redefined as more normal, or within a developmental frame; for example, as an understandable response to a difficult set of circumstances. Reframing conversations provide an opportunity to identify benign intent and positive motivation underlying a person's actions, such as the wish to protect self and others, or loyalty to family beliefs that may have outlasted their perceived usefulness. Reframes can emphasize the possibility for change by using active language rather than passive language, thus highlighting personal agency and choice in the use of "doing" language rather than in the use of "being" language. For example, "how did you decide ...?"

It is a fundamental tenet of any use of reframing that people may be more likely to acknowledge some personal agency and consider change if their behaviour or the underlying intention is framed more positively. Thus reframing is helpful if the reframe fits the context in which it is being used. Clearly, it would be unethical to reframe abusive behaviour, although when trying to help people change abusive patterns of behaviour, it may be helpful to understand actions in a wider context, without in any way diminishing a person's responsibility for such behaviour.

Using genograms

When thinking inter-generationally, either with an individual family member or a generational system, genograms are useful both as tools for assessment and as therapeutic interventions in their own right, much as some psychotherapists might use time-lines with individuals. A genogram is a visual diagram of a family tree, spanning three to four generations, in which relationships, significant events, and the family's social history are mapped. Genograms are used to help track the inter-generational transmission of family culture; that is, the set of beliefs, traditions, values, and myths that are thought to influence our perceptions, attitudes, and choices in our interpersonal dealings with one another. As a method of collating demographic information with life events, it is a quick assessment method. It has the added advantages of informing family members about their family history, helping to engage family members in a therapeutic relationship, and is potentially a task that helps settle both the therapist's and the family members' anxieties early in the therapy relationship. It can provide a rationale for change in the therapeutic work, such as changes in secrecy boundaries, and has the therapeutic potential for rejoining tasks, such as bridging difficult inter-generational boundaries, emotional cut-offs, and suspending conflict (McGoldrick & Gerson, 1989). Genograms can be used in a focused, therapeutic way. For example, using a genogram to trace a family history of separation and divorce as a way of understanding expectations of and attitudes to intimate relationships; or tracing the impact of illnesses and disabilities within an extended system as a means to explore attitudes and roles in relation to the care of others.

When constructing a genogram with family members, the following questions are helpful in both contextualizing current behavioural choices and patterns, and in exploring the emotional quality of family relationships as they change over time.

- What life-cycle events/transitions have been more difficult for your family? Why might that be?
- What resources have family members drawn on in their attempts to cope with change?
- What beliefs might be influencing attempts to cope with change?
- What are/were the most significant relationships for you? Why?
- What alliances and coalitions can you identify? Were they overt or covert?
- What has influenced your family members' sense of ethnicity? Who has been important in influencing ethnic identity in the family?
- What gender issues seem to have been important?
- Are there family secrets? What effect do you think they have had on family members?
- What has helped/hindered your development within this family?

Genogram notation

Where possible, use a large sheet of paper, with the opportunity to Sellotape together extra sheets should they be needed. As the genogram is a visual tool, it is important that it can be seen by all participants. Family members may well wish to take it home to complete it and add in further information after consulting with extended family and others. One therapeutic task that helps to address emotional cut-offs is the fishing trip, i.e. taking the genogram to speak to another family member about gaps in knowledge and memory.

There a number of different approaches to drawing genograms. The differences are less important than agreeing the consistent use of notation within your own team and with individuals and family groups who seek therapy and consultation. Genograms also bear some resemblance to eco-maps, often drawn during team and organizational consultation. The notation used may be similar, although hierarchy, communication patterns, and strength of relationships may be drawn within different schema; for example, the use of family and organizational trees, concentric circle models of organizational structure, and communication pattern charts.

When drawing genograms, women are usually represented by a circle, and men by a square. Often, ages and names are written in and on the shape. Significant dates and events may also be noted nearby, such as date of death, or cause of death, main employment, and so on. Those family members who have died are often represented with shaded shapes. Significant and more permanent couple relationships and marriages are represented with a solid line connecting the two adult shapes. If they have separated or divorced, this is usually represented with two short lines cross-hatching the main line, and often with the date of separation or divorce written below the line. You may write the date of cohabitation or marriage above the line. Sometimes a dotted line is used to represent an intimate but short-term liaison.

Children born to a relationship are shown in an inter-generational relationship by their positioning below the adult couple. Try to be consistent in representing the birth order of children, although you may wish to highlight some children and their intimate partnerships, and so on, from the rest of the sibling group by drawing them larger. Again, ages and names are usually written in the shapes or near them. Twins are represented differently, with a small connecting line, before they are joined to the sibling birth line. It is usual practice to represent miscarriages and still-born children, and terminations of pregnancy, unless there is an ethical reason not to do so. Adoption and fostering status for children and parents is also indicated. You may well include birth family information in the overall picture in these circumstances.

Most genograms contain three-generational information, sometimes four. Significant life events may be listed in the corner of the page or, if used with a team for consultation purposes, working hypotheses and service issues may be listed. Use different coloured pens to represent different kinds of information. Some genograms can be complex, and colour helps to trace and identify patterns. In particular, you may wish to represent the perceived nature of emotional relationships on the genogram; for example, emotional closeness and distance, chronic conflict, triangulation, and emotional cut-off, using structural symbols. In our practice, when working with violent behaviour in family relationships, we draw violence lines between the shapes representing family members, often indicating with an arrow head the direction of the violent behaviour.

Problem-solving approaches

Problem-solving approaches are both popular and tried and tested with practitioners of many orientations (Nelson-Jones, 1988). Systemic psychotherapists have given a systemic gloss to some of the more common approaches, making them relationally based, with the questions asked *interventive* in their own right (Weakland *et al.*, 1974).

Thus, traditional questions designed to track (a) the development of a problem, (b) previously attempted solutions, and (c) the losses and gains around change have been expanded.

1. For whom is it most/least a problem?
2. What solutions have you and others tried?
3. Who would know first that the problem was no longer a problem? Who would know last?
4. What would be the main gain of solving the problem for you? For others? Who would most welcome the change?
5. What disadvantages could there be in solving the problem? For you? For others? Who would least welcome the change?
6. What would be the smallest acceptable change? For you? For others?

The advantage for us in contextualizing our problem-solving conversations in these ways is that we *expand* the frame of the problem by widening the relational perspective on what might be contributing to the problem, what might be maintaining it, and by including the relational effects. This facilitates potential solutions in a way that reduces a sense of personal failure or blame for the client.

In this next section, we shall turn to some of the "solution-focused" approaches, which developed in parallel with the more strategic problem-focused approaches. In our view, these map well on to motivational interviewing techniques, taught on many clinical and counselling psychology courses, and used by other mental health practitioners, particularly in substance misuse services.

Solution-focused approaches

Motivational interviewing is a highly individualized approach to counselling, used widely in the addictions field, to help someone who is ambivalent about their drink or drug use to contemplate change and decide for themselves to change (Miller & Rollnick, 1991). The approach is directive and actively encourages the client to explore for themselves both the good things about their substance use and the less good things, some of which may be important concerns for the client. Discrepancies are amplified; for example, how we saw ourselves in the past and what we hope for the future, or seeing ourselves as a person versus seeing ourselves as a substance user, as these discrepancies can be a powerful source of personal motivation. Summarizing themes and juxtaposing them is the aim of the counsellor, constantly seeking to develop a person's motivation to change.

The systemic solution-focused therapies draw on some of these motivational interviewing principles and strategies in a very creative way (Miller & Berg, 1995). The focus is very much on solutions, or the seeds of solutions that are already happening, rather than on the problems *per se*. It is assumed that, whatever the problem, there are always exceptions. The therapist is interested in where the client wants to be, rather than where they might be now, psychologically speaking. Thus, small changes in a person's life can be extended and, pragmatically speaking, if something works, do more of it, and if not, do something different. The underlying philosophical principle is that change is always happening, no matter how stuck people think they are. The solution-focused view of resistance to change is that you only get resistance if you push in the direction the client does not want to go. Motivational interviewers do not encourage confrontational techniques either, similarly arguing that, strategically, the goals for the work must come from the client.

Some practitioners would say they adopt a solution-focused approach in much of their work, but, in keeping with the principle of this book that some ways of thinking and working can be helpful, we offer some suggested questions that you might use when trying to amplify and encourage an exception to the "problem" in your clinical work. Clearly, answers to questions are constrained by the nature of the question and the way in which it is asked, and systemically speaking, questions can be used to help make connections more visible and change seem more possible.

The *miracle question* is probably best known. Its strength is as a conversation opener when a person feels very stuck with a problem, and in our experience, can help fan the flames of hope that change can happen. Obviously the question does not stand on its own; the art of the therapist is in following the leads offered within the answer. So, asking, "If there was a miracle one night when you were sleeping and the problem was gone when you woke up, how would you know?", can be followed up with "How would your friends/family/employer know?" "Who would be most surprised?" and "How would they show it?", which widens the emotional and relational consequences for change. "What is happening in your life/family/job now that you would like to see continue?" enables a connection to be made with the possible replies to the miracle question.

Scaling questions are designed to seek exceptions to the problem and have been long associated with the solution-focused approach. They take many forms. For example, you can ask, "What is different about the days when you do not have the problem?" and expand the relational focus by further asking, "What are you/your family, etc. doing differently?" If no exceptions to the problem are acknowledged, you can ask, "When is it less severe, intense or shorter in duration?" "On a scale of 0–10, how would you describe the best day/the worst day over the past week?" "How do you know what sort of a day it is going to be? What do you/others do differently on these days?"

Moving into *action questions* is important for the development of a sense of personal agency. Action questions follow the questions designed to create expectations for change, and to seek exceptions to the problem. The leap from belief into action is a transition that many therapeutic approaches struggle to define. The following questions are designed to reinforce beliefs in personal agency, as a prelude to action, and use the active language voice rather than the passive voice. For example, noticing any change, no matter how small, since deciding to seek a referral and coming to the first appointment, "What changes have you noticed about the problem since making the appointment and coming here today?" "Are they the kinds of changes you would like to see continue?" Or, about any exception or diminution of the problem, "How did you get that to happen?" "Who else noticed that you did that?" "Have you had a similar difficulty in the past?" "How did you resolve it then?" "What will be the first sign that you are feeling good again?" "What will you be doing?" "What plans will you be making?" Future-oriented questions, as a way of looking beyond a present difficulty, are thought to help enhance personal motivation for change.

Language

Although apparently very action-focused, solution-focused approaches also pay detailed attention to the use of language in families and in the therapeutic relationship. Taking ideas from pragmatics, they argue that the use of language is extremely important in shaping how people act. Many of the core ideas derive from the work of Milton Erickson (Haley, 1973), Bateson (1980) and Watzlawick and colleagues (1967). They emphasized that communication is multi-faceted and contains implicit and explicit commands. So, for example, they pay attention to the way a parent or therapist might inadvertently use words, such as "why", "but", "you should", in ways that increase rather than decrease resistance to change. For example, an adolescent might justify himself by saying, "I've tidied my room", to the query about whether he is helping more around the house, to be met by the response "Yes, but you never help with the dishes". Perhaps less obviously, therapists can also fall into such resistance—making traps by directing a conversation away from statements about success to questions about the problem. In the context of eating disorders, for example, the conversation may shift from the young person saying she has successfully eaten something and is not feeling too bad, to questions about what the problems were about eating the rest of her meal. Solution-focused approaches pay attention to the specific details of how language may be employed and where such barriers to change may be erected.

The referral process and relationships with other agencies

A major systemic contribution to thinking about referrals and the complexity of the professional systems that can sometimes surround a family comes from the idea of exploring the history of coming for help before exploring the history of the problem.

The referring network

The cornerstone of the Milan systemic approach to family therapy has been in the definition of the professional network. In their paper "The problem of the referring person", published over twenty years ago, the Milan team outlined the development of their ideas about exploring the referring network around the family problem (Selvini-Palazzoli *et al.*, 1980a). Upon receipt of a referral they would hypothesize (a) about the interacting systems, (b) about the family problem, and (c) about the problem of the referring person within the network of agencies involved with the family. These hypotheses would then inform a plan of action.

The Milan team identified a number of recurring problems around failure to engage families in therapy. They concluded that in many of these cases they had failed to take into account the long-standing and homeostatic nature of the relationship between the family members and the referring person. For example, they observed that family members attended to please the referring person, because at all costs they wished to preserve this relationship. Thus, family members' engagement in therapy was cursory, either masked by courtesy or frankly hostile and complaining. In these cases the referring person might have been frustrated by their own failed attempts to help the family members make changes, or might have needed the family therapists to help them extricate themselves from an over-involved relationship with some of the family members, and so referred the family to therapy as a last-ditch attempt to help. In response to these referral and engagement difficulties, the Milan team would either invite the referring person to a family meeting so they could be well placed to continue the therapy subsequently, or they would construct an intervention for the family which included the referring person in an attempt to help the family decline therapy where it was not needed.

Networking and inter-agency practice

> There has not been very much written however, about how several systems inadvertently combine in their day-to-day operations in such a way as to frustrate each other's activities, and how, in so doing, they destroy in varying degrees the lives of people, or render it difficult for them to improve their lives. We have all been too tightly locked in our own niches by training, experience, and various types of private interest to see this kind of interlock ... [Hoffman & Long, 1969]

This quote was written in 1969. Writing over thirty years later, we think a similar description could apply to some of our work with families who have multiple relationships with professionals and agencies. In this section, we try to examine some of the complexity of working across agencies and explain how we believe systemic thinking can be helpful when participating in multi-agency network meetings.

Peter Hardwick (1991) provided a thorough and helpful analysis of network difficulties, actions of the professional network that can hinder change, and gave some pointers to dealing with network problems. He agreed with Skynner (1976) that family therapists and systemic thinkers need to identify the minimum sufficient network for intervention and recognize the influence of professional systems on families. Interestingly, this is not dissimilar to the notion of the "problem determined system" which emerged much later in the work of Anderson *et al.*, (1986). The term "multi-agency family system" was coined to describe the results of professional problem-solvers unwittingly joining the system they are trying to change and inadvertently helping it retain its coherence (Reder, 1986). When analysing the circumstances of a poorly functioning inter-professional system, Hardwick identified characteristics of the workers, the family members, and particular contextual features. Referrals are scrutinized carefully, in order to establish whether they are covert requests to take over the referrer's role, or the same request repeated through a series of workers. Hardwick is particularly alert for referrals where many agencies are contacted simultaneously. The parallels with the Milan team's paper described above are clear.

In collaboration with a group of colleagues, he went on to identify network difficulties when one or more of the following features are present in their work: (a) when the reason for the referral is not clear; (b) when the family does not attend the assessment appointment; (c) when a family thought to be well engaged in the therapy fails to attend a meeting; (d) when the referrer is asking for yet another assessment; (e) when recommendations following a clinical assessment are not implemented; (f) when other workers in the professional system describe family members as resistant; and (g) when the team is aware of pressure to act in powerful ways and perhaps take action inappropriate to their roles.

In addition, they outline ways in which actions of the professional network can hinder change, including their own and others' actions, such as: (a) network advance; (b) network retreat or abdication; (c) network freeze; (d) network over-protection; (e) scapegoating processes; and (f) multi-agency mirroring. Hardwick and his colleagues were well aware that as service providers they could also be part of the problem, so to speak, and that their attempts to be helpful could further block progress in effective communication and problem-solving.

"Network advance" is a way of describing what happens when professional workers take over responsibility for family members' behaviour, either by invitation or through a longer process of professional befriending. This would be an example of a complementary relationship between family members and professional workers that on the surface appears benign. As family members appear to seek dependency or behave in ways that raise professional anxiety about their abilities to cope, workers take on more responsibility for the family, thus inadvertently reinforcing family members' beliefs that they cannot cope well, or at least not without professional support. Such a pattern might be seen in family systems where each generation of parents and children are involved with the social services, which provides material, practical, and social support to the family. The tightness of the complementary fit can be seen to emerge at the level of belief systems, whereby the social support agencies might like to "do good", so to speak, and the family members might like having "good" done to them.

An example of network advance that appears hostile would be the symmetrical escalation seen when professional interest in a family or family member is perceived as a threat. This could lead the family members to try to retreat from professional scrutiny, which then raises network anxiety and suspicion and might lead to further escalation, resulting in a crisis intervention, such as emergency hospitalization for mental health concerns.

"Network retreat or abdication" can be seen when denial by the family members of the seriousness of the difficulties in the family is maintained and mirrored by similar processes of denial within the professional network. Passing the buck of responsibility for dealing with the issues of concern can happen within an agency—for example, waiting for a new colleague to start and take on the case—or between agencies. If a referrer presses the panic button and involves as many other agencies as possible, it is wise to ensure that responsibility is not diluted between agencies as a result. Deference may show itself in workers in one agency overestimating the skills and abilities of workers in another agency, or in justifying their lack of action while waiting for a response from another agency. Further dilution of responsibility within a professional network can occur in the network "huddle"—when a decision is made to hold yet another network meeting without any clear plan.

"Network freeze" describes the effects of professional workers who cannot agree on how to proceed, whereby their divided opinions serve only to cancel each other out, maintaining the status quo and inaction on the part of professional workers and their agencies.

"Over-protection" is a term used to describe prevailing beliefs within a professional network that putting pressure on a family will result in a crisis or a disaster, such that few expectations of family members' behaviour are articulated, and change is not facilitated. Some instances of adolescent behaviour, such as school refusal or deliberate self-harm, can lead to the development of complementary patterns within a professional/family network, fuelled by the tendency to over-protection in the face of significant anxiety.

"Scapegoating" within a network can result from feelings of inadequacy, confusion and frustration in response to lack of change, leading some professional workers or family members to blame each other, for example, "the family is not motivated", or "your colleague understands us better". Professional workers absent from a difficult network meeting might subsequently hear that they have been scapegoated. Finally, Hardwick draws our attention to multi-agency mirroring, through which professional workers and family members can replicate the role confusion, unresolved conflict, and distorted communication within their systems in an iterative manner. Reder (1986) has written of similar processes when describing the potential pitfalls of working with the "multi-agency family" system, with one professional from a different agency involved with each family member. Another example can be found in some adversarial child custody disputes, with professionals "splitting" along the divorcing couple's conflict fault-lines and taking up polarized positions with respect to each other and the "other side".

Hardwick offers some useful pointers to dealing with network problems, summarized as: (a) look before you leap; (b) map the system; (c) meet the system; (d) search for systemic patterns; and (e) try to reduce network problems. You will probably notice many similarities in this next section with the advice offered to systemic consultants by Wynne *et al.*, (1986), featured in Chapter Six.

"Look before you leap" is about thoughtfulness around the referrer and the referral. Such thoughtfulness can be promoted by asking a series of questions, of yourself, the referrer, and your clients. Thus, it is helpful to clarify who actually wants the referral, to ask why now, and ascertain who else is involved and how they may have become stuck, and to what extent expectations of you and your agency are clear. Has the referrer prepared the family members for the referral, does the referrer have a solution in mind, and is the referrer taking responsibility for their own ideas and actions in relation to your new relationship with the family members? In a similar vein, Reder and Fredman (1996) have written recently on their experiences of clients' relationship to help. We shall discuss their work later in this section; as it has many parallels with the ideas discussed here.

Many colleagues have said to us over the years that such thoughtfulness around the referral, while advisable, is too much of a luxury in the face of waiting lists and limited time and resources. We would agree to some extent, in that many of our referrals can be considered fairly straightforward. However, what experience teaches us is to identify early signs of network difficulties and try to deal with them before becoming embroiled in a confusing, complex, and potentially unhelpful piece of work. We hope this section goes some way towards alerting the reader to these signs in their own practice.

"Mapping the system" is essential in our view, whenever accepting a referral. This can be a brief process, which is updated regularly as you gather information and get to know people. It can involve sketching out the relevant system in your mind's eye on paper or in discussion with a colleague, or it can be raised in supervision, and so on. Alternatively, it can be a more detailed and formal process initiated through a network referral meeting and designed to clarify roles and responsibilities before embarking on a piece of work with a family, who themselves have multiple relationships with other professionals. Full network meetings are often advisable when you receive repeat requests for an assessment as a result of your previous conclusions not according with the views of the referrer. Chairing an initial network referral meeting with clarity, purpose, and an understanding of how complex systems interlock, is a crucial skill which contributes to the success of the work. Invitations to a network referral meeting would, ideally, include all relevant professional workers and family members. In practice this is often not achieved, so asking circular questions of the attenders about their views of what others might hope for and expect is a helpful way of including absent network members and keeping their presence alive in the room.

Mapping the system is an attempt to paint a developmental picture of the family and their difficulties, strengths, and resources. For example, determining who are the significant family members and others—from the household, community and extended family systems, including the professional system—the history of their relationships and, crucially, the system's relationship to the present referral. It may be that an attempted solution to the problem has become the problem (Watzlawick *et al.*, 1974). If so, track carefully what has been done to try to solve the problem, who else is working with the family, their attitude towards the referral, and ideas of what people are hoping for as a result of this referral, both from those attending an initial referral network meeting and those who are absent. Leave your options open if recommending an intervention following a network referral meeting. You might enquire about what the people present will do if you are unable to provide what they are hoping for, as well as what they think absent network members will do. Careful tracking of these views is usually fruitful, because the conversation often contains seeds of future solutions hidden in less preferred actions or unrealized resources.

"Meeting the system" overlaps with mapping the system. If a brief and early attempt to map the system uncovers information about a complex set of family/agency/professional worker relationships, it is helpful to try to convene the network to clarify professional roles and relationships so as to become a more effective helping system, in the manner described above. If the original reason for an agency's involvement with a family or other professional group has been long forgotten or has become unclear, asking the following questions can focus the network: (a) what is the problem now, as you see it?; (b) what is the history of your agency's involvement?; (c) what instigated this involvement? (a social worker will often compile a chronology of social work agency actions and concerns that can be very helpful in contextualizing current concerns); (d) what was done then?; (e) what are you doing now?; and (f) what is the aim of your work? Tracking overlapping and interlocking professional ideas and actions within a historical frame can offer clarity where little existed previously. The gentle art of reframing (Watzlawick *et al.*, 1974) is useful in identifying positive motivations and strengths in a context that may have been characterized by confusion and some blaming of others.

Thinking systemically on your feet in network meetings is a skill that develops with practice. In our early attempts at chairing such meetings, we found it helpful to be joined by a systemically-minded colleague as a co-chair, or in-room consultant, which allowed us to stay focused on the content of the meeting while not losing sight of important group systemic processes. Hypothesize about systemic patterns, such as the system and its rules, both explicit and covert, or where the competition occurs, i.e. who works best with the client. Consider whether some patterns can be changed. Think about the interaction of belief systems. For example, where family members are professional workers, how might that affect their view of the problem? What do we think the family members' hypotheses are about us, about the other agencies, and *vice versa*? Are there symmetrical or complementary patterns of fit?

When trying to reduce network problems, we can think of our own responsibilities and how we can use good supervision to help us understand the complexities involved. How do we think about ourselves and our relationships within our own families, and how might that indicate with whom we are most likely to identify, or avoid? What defences do we use, and what kinds of dilemmas, conflicts and anxieties might we encounter that triggers them? To what extent are we clear about our own professional role, our sources of influence, and the concomitant limits and responsibilities? And finally, it is important to know our own professional networks and how our role relates to that of others.

In summary, based on our experience, it is always helpful to ask the following questions of a referrer when accepting a referral of a family/client group lodged firmly within such a complex professional network:

- what is the history of your agency's involvement with this family/client group?
- what happened at that time to initiate your agency's involvement?
- what did you or your predecessors do at that time?
- what was the outcome?
- what is the problem now, as you see it?
- what are you doing now to help solve the problem?
- what is the aim of your agency's work?
- what are you/the family hoping for from me?
- what will your agency/the family do if I am unable to offer help?
- what will everyone else do if I am unable to be helpful?

- who else is working with this family/client group?
- do they know about your referral to me?
- what are their attitudes towards your referral?
- what do you think they are hoping for from me?

Asking these questions may well surprise a referrer/referring network, but creates a context for reflection around complex interagency referrals where the history of professional involvement may have given rise to ambivalence about the possibility for change for the better.

The relationship to help

Reder and Fredman (1996) have further developed previous contributions to systemic thinking and practice around the processes of referral. They are interested in what they have termed "the relationship to help" and how asking questions to elucidate this relationship can facilitate effective referral processes and help build good client/professional relationships. They assume that clients and professional workers hold beliefs about each other and the helping process itself which can exert a significant influence over engagement and treatment processes.

They encourage referrers to speak to them first on the telephone, and attempt to map the network of professional relationships linked to the referral (Hardwick, 1991). In this conversation, they explore the relationship between the client and the referrer, attempt to address the history of the client's relationship to helpers, and gather information about the client's and referrer's attitudes to referral. Particularly, they ask about the referrer's previous contact with them, such as, "Did anything happen then that might influence our liaison around this present case?" When they meet the client they map the client's expectations and view of existing relationships using similar questions. In particular, they have found that mapping the client's relationship to help and its basis in earlier relationships, including family relationships or beliefs, can have a helpful effect on their subsequent contact.

Reflexive notes

1. If you have not used a genogram before, we would strongly recommend that first you complete your own, with the aid of a trusted colleague, using the questions on page 42 to aid your exploration of patterns of relating in your own family. This will give you an idea of your clients' experiences of doing a genogram. It will also alert you to your significant inter-generational relationship themes and issues that may resonate when you construct genograms with clients, and so help prevent unhelpful mirroring.
2. You might like to interview yourself or a colleague around some everyday minor irritation, using some of the questions listed under problem-solving approaches (pp. 44–45). In the feedback, reflect on what you noticed about yourself in relation to the different questions.
3. Think of a minor irritation at work. Describe in detail what life will be like and what you will be doing differently when you are no longer experiencing this irritation. Reflect on what expectations of change were created as a result.
4. Where does your agency/team/service get stuck in its relationships with other agencies/teams/services?
5. How does your agency/team/service define itself in relation to its tasks? How do you think members of the public might define the key tasks of your agency/team/service? What do you think happens when respective sets of beliefs are in conflict?

CHAPTER THREE

Systemic formulation

Formulation in clinical practice

The skills of assessment and formulation have been fundamental in the development of many of the therapeutic professions. For example, from the start clinical psychology nailed its colours to the positivist traditions of science and promised to provide a rigorous and evidence-based approach to clinical work. In the early days of the profession clinical psychologists often worked alongside psychiatrists to provide detailed "objective" assessments, frequently employing standardized tests that shaped clinical formulation. The purpose of the assessments was largely to diagnose with accuracy deficits in functioning with the aim of clarifying their extent and nature. Once established, this was employed to indicate the direction of treatment. For example, a psychologist might assess the extent of impairment in a young child apparently demonstrating learning disability. Based on the assessment particular regimes of interventions might be attempted such as, behavioural programmes to improve the level of independence or communication.

We can propose that formulation is central to any therapeutic activity. It represents the essential link between theory and practice—how we view difficulties and how we intend to assist people and their families. The two main strands of formulation; assessment and treatment planning are intertwined. Every theoretical model can be seen to contain different ideas about what to look for in assessing a problem and subsequently how to treat it. Many mental health practitioners are encouraged to employ a variety of theoretical and treatment models; for example, combining relatively individual therapeutic approaches with systemic ones. Although many clinicians appear to find their own idiosyncratic ways of attempting such a synthesis, there has been relatively little provided in the way of systematic models to guide this integrative process.

As a consequence of a multi-model based training, therapists are faced with the task of attempting to be both *outside* and *inside* the models that they employ. This poses some difficult dilemmas; for example, an initial decision needs to be made about which model or combination of models should be employed in any given case. However, each model may contain discrete ideas about how to proceed with formulation and connections to other models. Arguably, this is particularly the case for systemic therapy. From *inside* a systemic perspective, it is argued that it offers an integrative model which allows us to include therapeutic work with individuals, and to work with parts of a family, the whole family, and other systems, such as school and work, and so on. However, from the *outside* this position can look like an act of faith or zealous commitment to one approach—systemic therapy. From the *outside*, systemic therapy represents one choice of model and, for example, is seen as having distinct features, such as the emphasis on pattern, meaning, and communication in relationships. This may be seen in contrast to, for example, a CBT approach which emphasizes a person's internal cognitions and representations of their experiences.

We will take a little space in this chapter to discuss these issues by looking relatively briefly at the question of the initial choice of a model. We will then consider how a systemic approach can be seen not as just another approach, but as one that encourages an integrative approach to clinical work.

Let us turn to a clinical example in order to start to explore some of the issues.

Case example: Charlie—a 15-year-old boy with suicidal and behavioural problems

Charlie was initially referred to the adolescent community service via his GP because he had become very withdrawn, was threatening to self-harm, was at times aggressive towards his mother, was using illegal drugs, was absent from school, and was displaying a variety of apparently psychosomatic symptoms. He came into contact with the Youth Offending Service because, with some friends, he had entered into neighbours' properties through the loft space.

Charlie was an only child living at home with his mother Sarah. His father (Brian) had committed suicide when Charlie was four years old and subsequently his stepfather (Nigel) died of a heart attack while Charlie was alone in the house with him. Charlie was nine years old at the time and it was apparent that both Sarah and Charlie were still upset at this loss. Sarah felt that she had lost control of Charlie and was extremely concerned that he might harm himself and come to a similar fate as his father. She felt unable to cope, appeared quite depressed, and seemed overwhelmed by Charlie's problems and behaviour. Sarah had a relationship with a younger man (Steve) who had been a friend of Nigel's son, Pete. Steve had previously lived with Charlie and Sarah, but Sarah had felt that he was too emotionally dependent and at times was like a second child rather than a father figure to Charlie. As Sarah attempted to develop some separation from Steve, he threatened to kill himself, and eventually engaged in a suicidal gesture by cutting his wrists at her home while she was out.

Sarah's parents lived close by and had become very involved in offering support to Sarah and in attempting to gain some control over Charlie's behaviour. Sarah's brother, Eddie, had his own family and occasionally was in contact with Charlie and Sarah. Charlie stayed with his uncle sometimes and usually "behaved quite well", though more recently he did not want to stay with his uncle. Sarah's parents had taken Charlie to live with them temporarily, to give Sarah some space to recover. However, they initially felt Charlie had a mental illness, perhaps like his father, that needed to be treated. This was later highlighted when, in an initial family assessment,

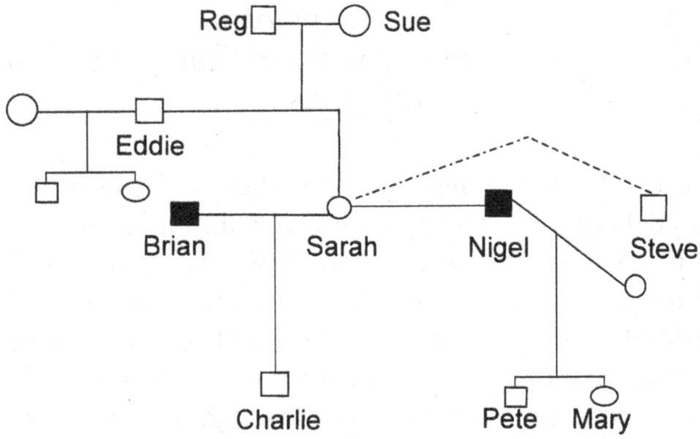

Figure 1.

Sarah's father (Reg) came to the meeting with the results of his searches of the Internet on a variety of psychiatric disorders: schizophrenia, ADHD, and Borderline Personality Disorder, which he felt fitted Charlie's symptoms!

Which model?

Relatively few integrative models have been produced. However, one comprehensive model has been developed by Weerasekera (1996), and this uses as a core axis a division between individual and systemic factors which are then explored in terms of their respective models of aetiology and their treatment implications (Figure 2).

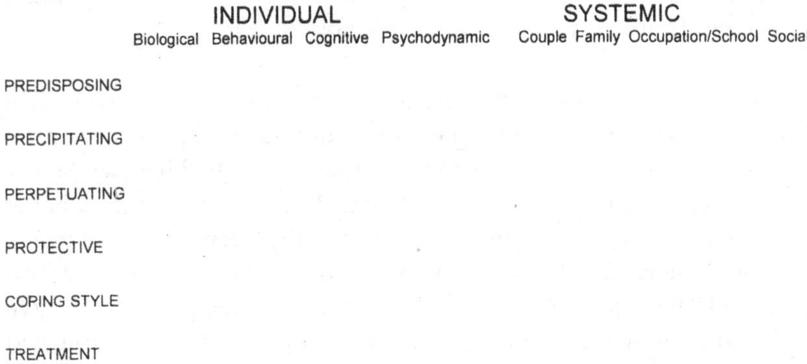

Figure 2. An integrated model of formulation. (From: Weerasekera, 1986.)

Individual versus systemic intervention

So, an initial decision suggested by this model is whether the problem might be approached most effectively from an individual versus a systemic perspective. Key to this initial decision is an assessment of the client's "preferred coping style" and this includes both the therapist's impressions as well as the client's expressed preference for forms of treatment. For example, a person may state that they do not wish their family members to be involved in the treatment of their problem. In practice the decision is far more complex; for example, in work with children it may be difficult for a child to articulate whether he or she wishes to attend with their family. It may also be the case that with many problems there is fairly convincing evidence that a range of relational issues are central, but facing these problems might prematurely raise anxieties and provoke avoidance of family work. There is a considerable tension, therefore, between the extent to which we can fully work collaboratively versus taking some charge or promoting a decision to engage in family therapy.

Weerasekera's (1996) proposed model attempts to deal with this thorny issue in part by focusing on what she calls "coping styles". The initial formulation therefore includes an assessment of the characteristic or preferred ways that the person has of coping with his or her problem. For example, some people express an initial preference to "understand" their difficulties but find it hard to address deeper emotional or relational issues. It is suggested that by accommodating to the person's initial style it is possible to strengthen the therapeutic relationship. However, as work progresses it may be possible that the client is able to risk extending the range of work to other forms of individual work or to systemic work. A thread running through formulation, therefore, is whether the various models are to be employed *simultaneously* or *sequentially*. We may decide, for example, that treatment might helpfully commence by the simultaneous application of a cognitive approach with a young person with anorexia and work with the family system. Alternatively, we may feel that a period of individual work might need to take place before progress with family work is feasible.

Why systemic?

It is possible to identify a number of factors that might suggest that a systemic approach is appropriate:

- there is indication of direct precipitative factors in the family, for example traumatic events such as bereavements, illness, or separations;
- there is clear evidence of relational difficulties within the family and/or between the family and other systems, such as the extended family;
- the client is aware of connections between his or her problems and relational issues in the family.

Returning to the example of Charlie and Sarah above, it was apparent that there was an initial belief that the problem was predominantly Charlie and that some individual work needed to take place. This belief seemed to be shared by Sarah and her parents and it seemed that to avoid this issue would have conflicted with the family's beliefs at that time. However, it also seemed clear that there had been some significant events in this family, such as the suicide by Charlie's father and the death of Nigel. It also seemed that Sarah was in a difficult relationship with Steve, and that the input from her parents to the management of Charlie may have had complex effects, for example, in making it harder for her to exert clear authority over Charlie.

It seemed that a helpful approach might be to start with some individually focused work with Charlie, exploring both medical questions and some of his feelings and beliefs, especially about the losses in his life and how these might be connected to his distress. This approach seemed to fit with Sarah and her parents' beliefs about what needed to happen. However, it also seemed that Sarah, in particular, recognized that there were historical and family issues that were relevant. She also demonstrated a psychologically-minded coping style in that she did see the value of discussing feelings, beliefs, and relationships. However, her parents were initially more concerned with a medical approach, seeking answers to the question of a diagnosis for Charlie. They also had a behavioural orientation, feeling that Charlie needed clear rules and discipline in his life. It was thought, therefore, that some initial therapeutic work focusing on Charlie and some clarification of his psychiatric status was necessary before other work, for example, family therapy, could take place.

Charlie was referred to the Adolescent Community Team. This consists of an integrated service which combines a number of workers who attempt to offer individual assessment and input, some involving home visits along with a systemic service comprising a weekly family therapy clinic. In addition, the service involves supervision of cases within a multi-model perspective. Typically, as in this case, there may be some initial tensions between the direction of work that the family and referrers may think is most appropriate and the beliefs of the team. In this case it was felt early on that family work was indicated and might become the main direction of work. In fact, Charlie seemed to endorse this view since he did not wish to engage in individual work following some initial sessions with the worker. However, the focus of the referral and requests from other agencies, such as the Youth Offending Service, indicated a focus on Charlie rather than the dynamics of the systems in which he was involved.

The politics of formulation

It is tempting to aspire to promote schemes of assessment and formulation that set out clear and detailed guidelines that clinicians might be able to follow. It may be helpful to contemplate developing such maps, not least in that efforts to produce them may reveal the complexity of the task involved. However, we suggest that formulation contains within it the core conceptual, psychological, and philosophical issues relating to therapy. Most fundamentally we are compelled to consider what we believe to be a problem or symptom. Related to this are questions about who is experiencing the problem: the person, the family and/or the community, and so on.

Arguably an important point of contrast between the psychotherapies and psychology on the one hand, and psychiatry on the other hand, is the relative weight given to formulation versus diagnosis. Simply, psychology tends to concern itself more with developing formulations of difficulties than engaging in attempts to diagnose or assign labels to constellations of difficulties. More specifically, psychology and psychotherapy has been closely concerned with debates about the relative merits of medical versus social models of problems. Taking a medical view assessment is largely about accurately establishing correct diagnoses of conditions. Formulation then follows in a relatively straightforward way, mapping out ways to manage or treat the diagnosed disorders.

Similarly, family therapy has been critical of medical models and instead offers a more social model of the causes and maintenance of problems. Significantly, it has also developed to be increasingly critical of medical and pathologizing processes (Dallos & Draper, 2000; Hoffman, 1993; White & Epston, 1990). Within this framework family therapy offers a critical position in that it endeavours to question the potentially oppressive assumptions that may be made about family members, and even that family members may have been conscripted into holding about themselves:

> I sometimes think that 99% of the suffering that comes in through my door has to do with how devalued people feel by the labels that have been applied to them or the derogatory opinions they hold about themselves. [Hoffman, 1993, p. 79]

In essence this is the cornerstone of the social constructionist (post-modern) position that characterizes the third phase of the family therapy movement. As with the psychotherapies more broadly, this places the clinician working with families in a variety of complex positions regarding formulation:

- as an employee of the state we may feel pressure to offer formulations which contain elements of social control, for example, to enable a child in a family to become "less disruptive" and return to school;
- we may be critical and sensitive in our formulations of patterns of inequalities and oppressions which have shaped the problems in the first place;
- we may be aware of the competing definitions of what and whether there is a "problem"—the individual's view, the family view, differences of opinions within the family, the view of various agencies, such as the police and social services, involved with the family, school, the legal system, cultural systems, and the therapist's professional system.

In effect a primary aspect of formulation is the juggling of these competing definitions or constructions regarding problems in families. For example, for a clinical psychologist engaged in family therapy there is a need to take account also of the legacy of clinical psychology and the expectations that other professional colleagues hold. Substantially there may be a set of expectations that clinical psychologists are "experts" at assessment and formulation and, more specifically, that they will be able to assess whether an individual in a family "really" has an individual versus a family-based problem.

Again with reference to Charlie, it is possible to see the influence of these wider issues in the work with him and his family. A range of pathologizing processes had come into play. For example, there appeared to be a belief not only in mental illness but also about its heritability, especially seen in the considerable concern expressed that Charlie was like his father. Brian was described as having been a drug user, violent, unstable, and eventually had committed suicide. This concern about mental illness significantly featured in the grandparents' views about Charlie and, to a lesser extent, in Sarah's views. However, it can be seen as part of a much wider discourse regarding the nature of emotional distress. The belief in a medical model was shared not only by family members but also by the family GP, by Charlie's school and, to some extent, the Youth Offending Service. Arguably, Charlie was one of the few people who were actively resisting this definition. When his behaviour became more outwardly directed rather than internally focused, for example, offending behaviour, it is possible that in a way he was trying to state that he was angry rather than mentally ill. An important issue, then, may be the extent to which work with Charlie, including the initial formulation of the problems, takes into account the wider socio-political contexts and attempts to challenge these (Boyle, 1990; Dallos, 1997; Johnstone, 1993).

Systemic formulation

In this section we want to retrace our steps and look at the development of formulation in systemic thinking, and to make some links with other approaches such as functional analysis.

Systemic family therapy contains several features in its orientation to formulation that are sympathetic to the practices of other mental health disciplines. These include the following:

- a holistic approach
- the use of "working hypotheses"
- a multi-dimensional approach
- integration of a variety of theoretical positions—a multi-perspective approach
- a critical and reflective orientation
- evidence-based orientation

In particular, we suggest that systemic theory offered a substantial development in its secondphase in the move from an "outside" and "expert" position to a constructivist view that acknowledged the subjective nature of knowledge and knowing.

Functional analysis and progressive hypothesizing

Increasingly, the level of sophistication and the nature of assessment and formulation has progressed. Many mental health practitioners now would not attempt only an assessment of the individual in terms of his or her abilities and experience but also would look holistically at the various contexts in which the person was immersed. A considerable conceptual development in assessment and formulation has been inspired by behavioural analyses—the ABC model—antecedent–behaviour–consequences. Such an analysis focused on the factors that triggered behaviours/symptoms and the factors that subsequently maintained these. An extension of this form of analysis came to be called "functional analysis". This broadened a strict behavioural analysis to include "internal" events such as thoughts and feelings. For example, a functional analysis might suggest that one factor in the maintenance of aggressive behaviour is that it fosters a feeling of "power and retribution for perceived injustice".

The notion of the "function" of a problem or symptom also played an important role in psychodynamic thinking; for example, that amnesia might be functional in helping a person to avoid unbearable painful traumatic memories. However, "functional analysis" offered some significant developments.

- The function of a symptom was seen as related to secondary gains, such as the rewards that might be derived from the person's social context.

- Functional formulations were phrased in ways which made them subject to exploration and testing—they were refutable.
- By effecting alterations in the functional relationships, change was seen as possible in a relatively rapid way.

Importantly, "functional analysis" stressed both an intra- and interpersonal level of analysis. For example, an analysis of anorexia (Slade, 1982) proposed that the person might gain a perceived benefit by feeling more in control of their lives and proud of their ability to exercise control. In addition they might gain a perceived benefit by both gaining attention from their parents and indirectly offering a protest about the nature of their relationships. This move to an interpersonal analysis was important and offers significant links to systemic thinking.

> As an example, it could be proposed that Charlie's behaviour had been functioning to protect the family from the grief that had been experienced. Two traumatic deaths were very difficult for this family to deal with and the unbearably painful feelings were in a way avoided by the focus on Charlie's behaviour.

Assessment of family structure and process

As we saw in Chapter 1, systemic theory and practice has developed through a number of significant phases. In the first phase, as in early positivist and behaviourally inspired psychology, the emphasis was on making "objective" and "scientific" assessments and formulations. The family was seen as an entity "out there" that could be accurately described and assessed. The purpose, in large part, was to be able to map the nature of the dysfunction and subsequently to develop interventions to correct these. As with clinical psychology a range of standardized tests measuring family function were developed (Circumplex Model—Olson, 2000; McMaster model—Epstein *et al.*, 1993). In short, the aim was to assess dysfunctions of family structure and process. As an example, a family might be seen as having a lack of a clear hierarchy and decision-making capacity in the parental sub-system. Alternatively, they might be seen as caught up in a process whereby attempts by either parent to take control would be met by the other parent siding with the child. Once the problems were identified, the therapist working within an expert framework, would adopt interventions to alter them (see Chapter 1).

Function of a symptom

A cornerstone of early Milan-team systemic thinking was that symptoms in families served a *function* of stabilizing a family system. In many ways this appeared a counter-intuitive idea, since the established view was that the symptoms were the very thing that was causing the distress and unhappiness in the family. Jackson (1957) was the first to state clearly that a family with serious problems *could be seen as* a rigid or homeostatic system. Examples of this could be seen in accounts of how the removal of a patient from a family into psychiatric services could be followed by another member of the family developing some difficulties *as if* to maintain the status quo of the family dynamics. The classic example came from work with children where it was suggested that, for example, symptoms shown by a child could serve a *function* of distracting attention from the parents' conflicts with each other and thereby stabilizing the marriage. As the child's symptoms grew more intense the definition of the situation as the child having or being the problem would be reinforced. Functional analysis as developed by Slade (1982) put forward the notion of members of a family acting as if they had an investment in keeping the symptomatic member in that role despite overtly stating that they wanted them to change. Part of the functional analysis, therefore, was the extent to which a symptom in one member was meeting the needs of other members of the family and preserving the family *homeostasis*.

Attempted solutions

One of the most enduring and helpful ideas from the first phase is the model of formulation proposed by the Mental Research Institute (MRI) team. This consists of the elegantly simple idea that many problems arise from the failing solutions that are applied to ordinary difficulties; that is, the solution to the problem has become the problem (Figure 3). In this method of formulation the focus is on

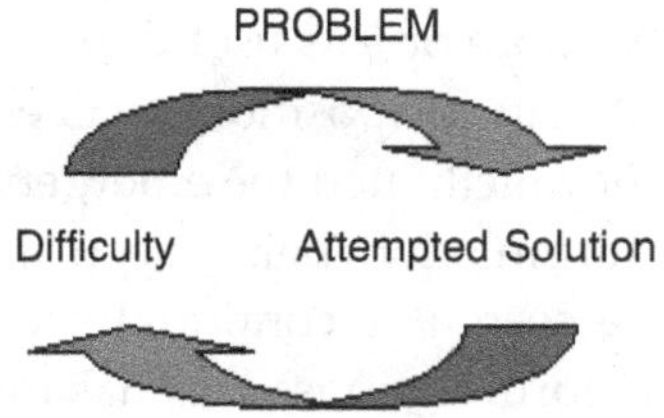

Figure 3. Model of formulation developed by the MRI team.

an identification of what is seen as the problem and how this is linked to difficulties that the family has attempted to overcome. The formulation consists of the following steps.

- Exploration of the problem.
- Deconstruction of the problem—when did it start, who first noticed, what was first noticed.
- Linking the problem to ordinary difficulties.
- Exploration of what was attempted to solve the difficulties.
- Beliefs about the difficulties and what to do about them.
- Discussion/evaluation of what worked/what did not work.
- What decisions were made about whether to persist with the attempted solutions and which solutions to pursue.

As we can see, this model bears a resemblance to functional analysis (ABC) in that attempted solutions in effect represent B behaviours, C consequences are the effects of the attempted solutions, and A antecedents are essentially the difficulties or triggers that set off the attempted solutions. Like functional analysis, this model assumes that there is a recursive cycle in play so that the attempted solutions can serve to construct a vicious cycle whereby there is an escalation of the difficulties.

The second phase of systemic family therapy saw a move towards constructivism. As we have seen, this stressed a view of reality as subjective. Families were no longer seen as "out there" nor the task of the therapy team as being to accurately assess their dysfunctional patterns. It was thought that we could only see a family through our own personal lenses. Consequently our descriptions and formulations were seen as having an "as if" quality—they were propositions rather than truth. As such these propositions could be more or less useful in guiding our work with a family. The value of our propositions was essentially in terms of the extent to which they facilitated the emergence of change. Instead of assessment and formulation being seen as a one-off scientific activity, it came to be seen as a continual process of developing—testing—and revising formulations. This has much in common with George Kelly's (1955) notion of "man the scientist"—that the essence of science and human experience is similar in that both are engaged in a process of enquiry in which ideas about the world are formed—tested—and revised where necessary (Dallos, 1997; Hoffman, 1998; Procter, 1996).

Progressive hypothesizing

> By hypothesising we refer to the formulation by the therapist of a hypothesis based upon the information he possesses regarding the family that he is interviewing. The hypothesis establishes a starting point for his investigation as well as verification of the validity of that hypothesis based upon scientific methods and skill. If the hypothesis proves false, the therapist must form a second hypothesis based upon the information gathered during the testing of the first. [Selvini-Palazzoli *et al.*, 1980a, p. 4]

The concept of punctuation was incorporated by the Milan team (Selvini-Palazzoli *et al.*, 1978) into the idea of therapy as inevitably progressing through a process of hypothesizing. There could be no objective truth about a family, simply our subjective perceptions as observers. The best we could achieve, therefore, was to formulate hypotheses (hunches) about what was going on that could be more or less helpful in our ways of working. This view broadly encapsulates the pragmatic position of the MRI group in that communication needed to be considered not just in terms of what was intended to be communicated but what its consequences were. Hence, a hypothesis was to be judged in terms not of its ultimate truth or falseness but of how effective it was in facilitating some positive change.

Constructivist approaches have repeatedly drawn attention to the fact that family members may disagree, sometimes violently, about their explanations and narratives. These have been seen as essentially interpersonal disagreements or struggles over the punctuation of events. More recently, this has been discussed in terms of the competing stories family members hold and which define previous and future events. The analysis of questions about the meaning of a problem, or symptoms, is similar to the processes of deconstruction employed in the analysis of literature and the social sciences. Deconstruction involves taking constructs apart, analysing and tracing their historical origins, examining their inner logic, exploring their contradictions and inconsistencies, exploring the situations that concepts are employed in, and considering what implications there are for action. When we engage in this process with families it is not unusual to find that the conflicts are not so much about disagreements as about different uses of a concept. Deconstruction can be employed as an activity that invites alternative meanings to be considered that by opening up the definition of a concept, can encourage, or at least lay the groundwork for, some mutually acceptable definitions to emerge.

The Milan team argued that the process of developing hypotheses was not only fundamental to the process of formulation but also to the practice of clinical work. They argued that the start of therapy with a family could be an extremely confusing affair and it could be easy for a therapist to feel overwhelmed by the amount of information that a family could present. A hypothesis could help to cut through this potential chaos and help to organize the information into a meaningful and manageable structure. Holding a clear hypothesis can help the therapist actively to engage the family by pursuing issues and asking questions to explore and test the hypothesis. This can serve to offer a direction to the work and help avoid the risk of simply floundering and perhaps unwittingly getting caught up in, or even aggravating, the family's problems. It can also help to reduce the anxiety of the initial contact (which can be considerable for all concerned, not least the therapist). A hypothesis was not to be seen as necessarily true, but as being more or less useful. A core aspect of this was the extent to which the hypothesis was elaborative, that is, it helped to elicit new information. The team went on to note a number of other important aspects of this process:

- explicitly forming and stating our hypotheses can help to reflect on our implicit assumptions which, if left implicit, may get in the way of therapeutic progress;

- articulation of hypotheses can help to reveal differences and agreements within the therapy team which again might impede therapy if left unstated;
- there is less pressure on the therapist to "get it right" which can reduce anxiety, especially in the early stages of therapy;
- as the engagement with the family is less of an "expert" position it may make it easier for the therapist and the team to remain curious and interested as opposed to trying to develop a correct formulation.

In practice there seemed to be times when the Milan team wandered from a constructivist position to making statements about their hypothesis being "correct" or "hitting the nail on the head". There was also a sense that the hypotheses were not always formed in a collaborative way with families.

Exploration of meaning and explanation

Arguably, the work of the Milan team also represented a significant move in that the focus of the hypotheses and formulations was concerned with the construings of the family members. Increasingly the emphasis was on the meanings that family members ascribed to each other's actions. For example, they describe a case of an adolescent boy who was displaying delinquent problems. The boy was living alone with his "attractive" divorced mother. Their first hypothesis was that his behaviour was intended to draw his father back into the family. However, they argued that this was rapidly disproved and it became clear that a more *accurate* hypothesis was that:

> The mother was an attractive and charming woman, and, perhaps after these years of maternal dedication, she had met another man, and perhaps her son was jealous and angry, and was showing this through his behaviour. [Selvini-Palazzoli *et al.*, 1980a, p. 4]

A proposed model of systemic formulation

We want to offer our own synthesis of approaches to formulation in systemic therapy and suggest that this can be summarized in a five-part model.

1. The problem—deconstruction.
2. Problem—maintaining patterns and feedback loops.
3. Beliefs and explanations.
4. Emotions and attachments.
5. Contextual factors.

As we have suggested, family therapy has moved through a number of phases and these significantly reflect the nature of the process of formulation. The phases have seen a shift from an emphasis on patterns and processes, on cognitions and finally on language and cultural contexts. These phases are also reflected in the scheme for formulation that has been proposed by Carr (1999):

1. repetitive problem—maintaining behaviours;
2. constraining belief systems and narratives;
3. historical, contextual or constitutional factors.

By the latter he is referring to factors such as family scripts, economic and social support and, importantly, the prevailing cultural values and norms.

Our proposed scheme shares many features of this model but we offer some additional points of focus. In addition, we suggest that it is important to think about assessment and formulation in terms of two interconnected processes: analysis and synthesis:

> *Analysis*: this entails exploration with the family of the nature of their family, each other, and their problems. Though it features in the early session this continues throughout therapy.
>
> *Synthesis*: this may follow or run alongside the assessment and analysis. It involves starting to integrate the strands of information into preliminary hypotheses or formulations of the problem.

This distinction between analysis and synthesis is consistent with a constructivist view which regards observation and gathering of information as an "active", "selective", and "interpretative" process. In starting to analyse the problem we are inevitably making assumptions and interpretations, for example, about what evidence is relevant, what further material we need, selectively attending to some factors and less to others. In recognizing this it may be possible to adopt a reflexive stance and be less vulnerable to becoming limited by our implicit assumptions.

1. The problem—deconstruction

The initial starting point from any therapeutic perspective is to explore the "problem/s". This involves a number of related questions:

- how is the problem defined: this includes further questions about whether the problem is framed predominantly as individual or interpersonal;
- how the problem affects relationships;
- how relationships affect the problem;
- for whom is the problem most difficult? Parents, siblings, people outside of the family, etc.;
- life history of the problem, when it started, how it developed, what factors influenced its development.

Exceptions

In the analysis of the problem it is also important to consider not only when and how the problem is seen to function but also to map strengths, and exceptions or "unique outcomes". These are times when the family has been successful in resolving the problems or can draw from other aspects of the wider family network to develop stories of competence, success, and so on:

- recent cases of success in overcoming the problem or when it has been absent;
- distant exceptions;
- exceptions in the wider family network;
- hypothetical exceptions.

> Sarah: described the problem as Charlie acting in destructive and, at times, aggressive ways towards her. However, the emphasis was also on her worries, that is, that part of the problem was how anxious she became about Charlie's well-being and in particular her concerns that Charlie might harm himself or ruin his life.

Charlie: appeared largely to deny that he had any problems and could not see what all the fuss was about. In particular he stated that he was staying off school because he did not like it and that he only used drugs to the same extent as other young people his age. He also believed that his mum had a problem in that she worried too much.

Grandparents: saw the problem as essentially residing in Charlie and that he was possibly demonstrating signs of serious mental illness which might lead to his coming to harm. They also saw the problem in terms of the effects it was having on Sarah—that she was depressed, stressed, and becoming physically ill.

Professional systems: Charlie's adolescent worker saw the problem in terms of Charlie's mental health and the potential risk of self-harm. The Youth Offending Team focused on the offending aspects of the problem and had to deal with the consequences of Charlie's actions on the community, especially his neighbours, whose property he had entered with his friends.

Exceptions: Alongside the description of the problems there were instances of actions that were indicative of competencies and health. For example, there were examples of Charlie being kind and considerate to his mother, of his intelligence and creative abilities at school. These were confirmed by the school. There was also an example of Charlie having heroically arrested a man who had threatened staff and stolen goods from a local store.

2. Problem—maintaining patterns and feedback loops

- Structures—exploration of the organization of the family. In particular this is concerned with mapping the family in terms of boundaries, power, and interconnected systems.

  In Charlie's family it is possible that Sarah's power as a parent was somewhat undermined by her parents who, in "helping her out", had also in effect taken over. Similarly, Sarah's relationship with Steve in some ways resembled having another son rather than a parental father figure for Charlie.

- Process and feedback loops—this emphasizes the exploration of repetitive patterns of behaviour based upon feedback loops between different parts of the system. One pattern that appeared to be present was between Charlie and Sarah:

> Sarah is concerned that Charlie is mentally ill and vulnerable like his father, but at the same time is anxious, stressed, and angry at his behaviour. She therefore monitors Charlie's actions and feelings closely, attempts to confront Charlie but then backs off, tired and tearful.
>
> Charlie feels he is being watched and that he is not trusted, and that he is seen as unstable. He responds in angry ways but also becomes ill, tired, and tearful.

In effect the more Charlie is distrusted the more he appears to act out and the more he acts out the more Sarah distrusts and is worried by his behaviour.

3. Beliefs and explanations

This part of the model invites exploration of the meanings that different family members hold regarding the problems and what should be done about it:

- Family beliefs
- Extra-family beliefs
- Socio-cultural beliefs and discourses
- Family members' perceptions, beliefs

> Connected to the above example, it seemed that a dominant belief was that Charlie has inherited a form of psychiatric illness similar to that of his father. At the same time there were beliefs that Charlie was suffering from delayed grief over the losses that he had experienced. Related to this, his mother, Sarah, appeared to believe that she was at fault for what Charlie had been through. At the same time Sarah also oscillated between feeling angry with Charlie and believing that he was being difficult and did need a firm hand. His grandparents (especially grandfather) seemed to hold these beliefs more extremely, feeling that they needed to offer some discipline but worried that Charlie was seriously ill. They also felt that Sarah was too soft with Charlie, and with people generally, and that Charlie needed a man to sort him out. For her part Sarah, though

appreciating the help her parents offered her, also resented that at times they treated her like a child—a feeling that she had harboured for many years prior to the current problems. The grandparents also felt that it was inappropriate for Sarah to be with a young boyfriend who was in competition with Charlie for affection rather than able to offer stability for him.

4. Emotions and attachments

Here, the nature of the emotional dynamics are explored, especially the attachments and emotional dependencies between family members and across the generations.

It appeared that there had been two traumatic losses in Charlie's family—Charlie's father and stepfather. It also seemed that there had been mixed emotions about his natural father, Brian, who had been unstable and at times violent. Consequently, Charlie's mother, Sarah (and her parents), may have found it difficult to share Charlie's grief at the loss of his father. With these feelings unresolved, the family then experienced a second traumatic loss that probably also affected Nigel's previous family. Consequently, both Charlie and his mother had lost central attachment figures and sources of love and support. In part, this may have shaped the system so that at times there was a role reversal, with Charlie having to look after his mother's emotional needs and her parents stepping in to take charge. This perhaps led to Charlie worrying about his mother and feeling that his mother could not look after him.

5. Contextual factors

At this point resources, history of the problem, environmental factors, extended family, role of professional agencies, and cultural discourses are considered.

Sarah was a single parent with relatively limited financial resources and her health was deteriorating. The pressures to work and provide for herself and Charlie, along with the worries she had about Charlie, combined to make her feel drained and stressed. She repeatedly stated that at times she felt so ill that she just could not cope with any problems and stress related to Charlie. She had to withdraw to her bedroom.

There had been a history of traumatic losses in the family and one aspect of this was the loss of a father for Charlie—both his birth father and stepfather, to whom he had been close. The family can also be seen as being in an important transitional phase, with Charlie becoming adult and facing the tasks of developing an adult identity and separation from his mother. It seemed that Charlie and Sarah had been through a lot together and may have found it difficult to negotiate some separation. Charlie's behaviour served to keep his mother highly involved with him and, for example, his absence from school also meant he spent more time at home with his mother. In turn, the involvement of the grandparents seemed to keep Sarah highly connected to her parents. At times she felt this was intrusive, for example, their disapproving attitude and advice about her young boyfriend.

Charlie and his family appeared to be caught up in a classic mad/ bad cycle within the various agencies. Charlie had been involved with child mental health services, social services and, on the other hand, with the police and the Youth Offending Service. Between them, the agencies found it hard to decide whether Charlie was "ill" and in need of therapeutic or medical input or criminal and in need of control and sanctions.

One dominant discourse in play was that of "mental illness". Apart from the diagnosis of the problem having the implication that the problems resided in Charlie, there are a connected set of assumptions and beliefs within this discourse:

- Mental illness is hereditary.
- Treatment requires medical methods, such as medication.
- Psychological factors, such as relationships in the family and traumatic events, are marginalized.
- A reflexive position is discouraged, avoiding the need for the other family members to explore their potential roles in the evolution of the problems and, importantly, risking not being able to recognize their own resources and competencies in the face of the problem.

Other less obvious discourses could also be seen to be relevant. For example, Sarah's parents perhaps disapproved of her having a younger man as a partner since this challenged the traditional family pattern of a woman supported by an older man. Moreover, Steve was financially insecure and more likely to be dependent on Sarah than to be a provider. At times this discourse prompted discussions in the therapy team of their own assumptions and prejudices that were not unrelated to the gender of the team members!

Synthesis: a systemic formulation

The above framework may help to direct our attention to the complex web of factors that have shaped and maintained the problem/s. However, it is easy to see that even the brief examples we have offered regarding Charlie and Sarah can quickly come to appear like an overwhelming kaleidoscope of factors. Somehow, this mass of information needs to be combined into a manageable formulation. This requires that we engage in a process of selection of what is seen to be key as opposed to peripheral to our understanding of the problem. In effect, this can be seen as an example of a fundamental psychological process—the construction of a narrative that embraces events, actions, and contexts into a story or "pattern that connects". The Milan team initially referred to this as "hypothesizing" but, as we saw earlier, this was in the sense of seeing a hypothesis as an attempt to construct frameworks of meaning rather than to objectively test the real causes of the problems in a family.

Progressive hypothesizing/formulation

The Milan team (Selvini-Palazzoli *et al.*, 1980b) emphasized that hypotheses should be seen as propositional and changeable. As we continually learn more about the family, we need to be able to revise our hypotheses so that we do not become blinkered by our preferred formulation.

Reflexivity

A systemic approach emphasizes the notion of the "observing" position and that the therapy system has its own dynamics and beliefs. It is important, for example, to try to be open to how our own family experiences may be colouring how we see a particular family or the actions of some members. Similarly, current life events in the team members will inevitably have a significant effect on our perceptions and formulations.

Collaborative approach to formulation

Systemic formulation has progressed, as has formulation more broadly in the psychotherapies, towards a collaborative, as opposed to an "expert" and outside, approach. Rather than seeing the family as an object about which we formulate, we can see ourselves as entering into a relationship with a family wherein we explore the problem/s and negotiate a shared formulation. This recognizes that it is not a prerogative of family therapists and psychologists but is an essential human activity, albeit the family's formulations may be less formal and shaped by specialist psychological language. If the family has a significantly different formulation to ours it is unlikely that therapy can take place.

Engagement—joining and the therapeutic alliance

The most clearly established common factor that determines how helpful therapy is likely to be is the strength of the therapeutic alliance (Pinsof & Catherall, 1986). A key ingredient of forming a strong therapeutic alliance appears to be that clients and families are able to develop "trust" in the therapist and the team. Related aspects are: (a) family members wish to "feel listened to", (b) that their "views are taken into account"; and (c) that the therapist is experienced as warm and non-critical. This suggests that the therapy system should be "authentic", and for example, not attempt to disguise significant differences in opinions and formulations about the problem/s. In our work, we attempt to discuss our evolving hypotheses with families in order to bring differences of opinion out into the open in an attempt to construct some agreed directions to the work. We should note that many families appear vulnerable and confused about their own formulations and it can be tempting to attempt to "help clarify" things for them. However, this can result in subsequent impasses when the family's core beliefs re-emerge.

Formulations: Charlie and Sarah

We offer some examples of potential systemic formulations of this case. None of these claims to be exhaustive but each attempts to offer a view that fits with the available information. In practice, this means that some features or details may be given more attention than others.

1. Charlie's problems were connected to the experiences of losses in the family. Not only had there been two important deaths of the fathers in the family but there had been mixed emotions about Charlie's birth father, which made it difficult for Charlie and his mother to communicate about their feelings. Sarah had become stressed, and her inability to offer strength and support to Charlie led to his confused behaviours. This drew attention from his mother but escalated as she grew increasingly desperate and hopeless. In turn, Sarah was becoming more concerned, but this alternated with anger and criticism of Charlie's behaviour. Sarah felt anxious about expressing her anger or setting boundaries for Charlie because she was worried that he might be vulnerable, like his father, and harm himself. This can be seen as a feedback loop (Figure 4).

This formulation views both Charlie and Sarah as having problems, and that this is related to an escalating process between them.

A related feedback loop is that Sarah's parents, at the same time as "helping", fuel a process whereby she feels increasingly inadequate as a parent and her parents feel increasingly compelled to intervene in order to "help" her.

2. Sarah is currently involved with a younger man who was a friend of Nigel, Sarah's second husband. This may have the effect of continuing to trigger the unresolved grief surrounding the losses. More specifically, it may be that Charlie's relationship

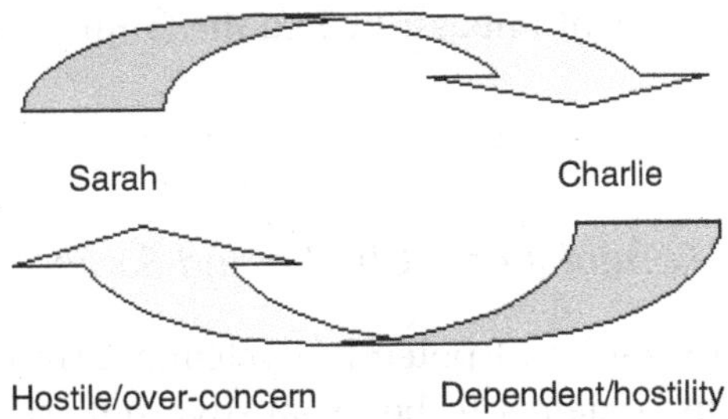

Figure 4. Mutually maintained pattern: Sarah is both angry and concerned, and is alternating between becoming over-involved with Charlie and withdrawing from him. Charlie is angry, but also feels vulnerable and dependent. He alternates between rejecting and being dependent.

with Steve is difficult, that Charlie feels displaced by Steve, and that he has to compete with him for mothering from Sarah. It is also possible that Charlie's relationship with Steve is confusing for Sarah since Steve is nearer to Charlie in his life-cycle, tastes, interests, and so on than Sarah. At times Charlie and Steve may be more like mates. This in turn may make it difficult for Sarah to exert any parental control over Charlie, and to involve Steve in this may be very confusing. As an example of these confusions we can speculate that it would be difficult for Charlie to explain to his friends the composition and nature of his household and his relationship with Steve. Also, Sarah embarked on the relationship with Steve at a time of distress and this set up a pattern of dependency between them. However, as Sarah became less dependent Steve became insecure and also resentful that he had previously looked after Sarah. For her part, Sarah was ambivalent about her relationship with Steve and sought contact with him when she felt vulnerable. Sarah and Steve needed to renegotiate the basis of their relationship but this was difficult because of Charlie's behaviour. This can be viewed as a triangular process (Figure 5).

Related to the triangular process Sarah's parents disapprove of Steve, and their views may impact on Charlie so that he feels confused and caught between his mother, Steve, and his grandparents (Figure 6).

Arguably, some of the contradictions above are also related to

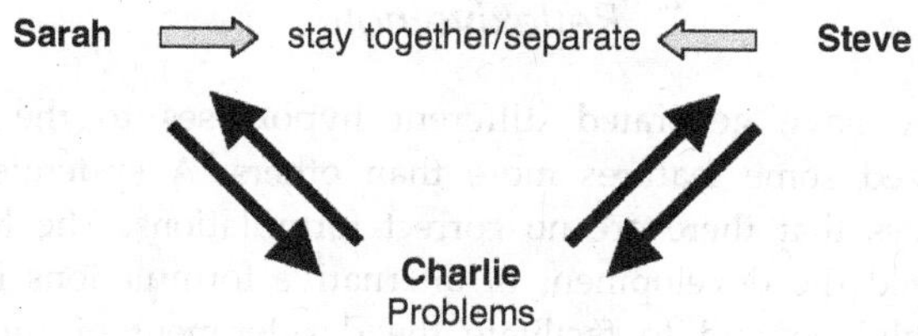

Figure 5. A triangular process. At times Charlie may have been seen as the cause of Sarah and Steve's problems at other times as suffering distress from their difficulties.

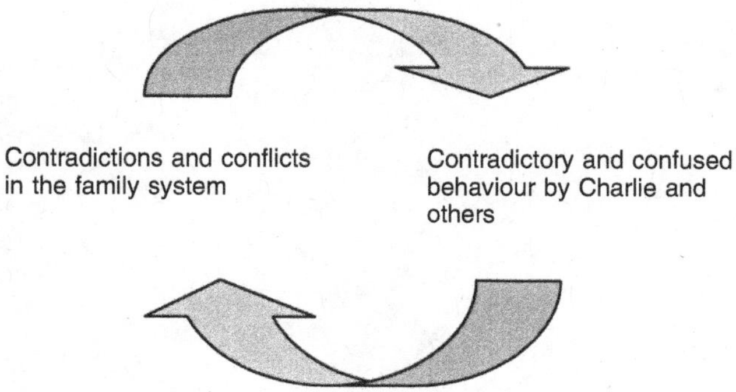

Figure 6. Further effects of conflicting views in the family.

shifting culturally—shared ideas about relationships, especially the role of men and women and family life. Sarah held more "modern" views of family life, as opposed to the more "traditional" views held by her parents. In becoming dependent on her parents she was subject to the influence of discourses that she had resisted in the process of separating from her parents as a young woman.

Reflexive note

1. You may have generated different hypotheses to the above, or emphasized some features more than others. A systemic approach emphasizes that there are no correct formulations. The Milan team encouraged the development of alternative formulations in order to clarify thinking and to facilitate the development of further, more comprehensive, formulations.

CHAPTER FOUR

Integrative practice: research on process and outcomes

In this chapter we shall overview some of the helpful findings from family therapy process and outcome research, as the empirical base for family therapy and systemic practice.

Does family therapy work?

This question is often asked by clinical managers who may be worried that a systemic approach will be too expensive to implement. The straightforward answer is yes, it does work, and the cost effectiveness advantages of family based interventions are beginning to emerge from a few studies. For example, Pinsof & Wynne (1995) review preliminary data that indicate family therapy is more cost effective than alternative interventions for adult alcohol problems and adolescent substance misuse. It seems that family therapy is more cost effective than standard in-patient and residential treatment for people with a diagnosis of schizophrenia and severe adolescent conduct disorders and delinquency.

Bergin and Garfield (1994) assert that the marital and family therapies have been subjected to rigorous scrutiny, with only a few other models of psychotherapy studied as often. The outcome literature typically reviews the couple/marital and family therapies together. Outcome studies have reported the use of controlled and uncontrolled group comparison designs across different psychotherapy modalities, single case designs, and outcome studies that compare the relative efficacy of different schools of family therapy. The findings from the research reviews and the meta-analytic studies are that family therapy works compared with untreated control groups, with some demonstrated superior effects over standard and individualized treatments for some psychological problems and groups of people (Pinsof & Wynne, 1995). The meta-analytic studies show moderate, statistically significant effects, and often with clinically significant effects. The research literature in support of these conclusions is as robust as it is for the other modes of psychotherapy studied as often (Carr, 2000a,b; Cottrell & Boston, 2002).

To start with, we need to consider a little of what we mean by "does family therapy work?" In family therapy, this question immediately has a number of strands:

(a) is there significant change in the person who has been identified as having the problem;
(b) is there change in other members of the family;
(c) is there overall change in the family dynamics and organization?

In systemic therapy, the "problem" is not seen to reside in any one person, yet obviously outcome needs to take account of the initial presentation. However, it is worth noting that back in the 1950s, Jackson (1957) pointed out that positive change in one member of a family is frequently accompanied by deterioration in another. He called this maintaining the status quo, or homeostasis, so that overall, the level of distress within the family group stayed the same. So, when comparing family therapy to individual based treatments, this aspect of an overall systemic evaluation also needs to be borne in mind.

A second set of questions relate to what we regard to be "change". Broadly, we would classify aspects of change as:

(a) behavioural;
(b) cognitive/beliefs;
(c) emotional.

This is the traditional tripartite view but is relevant to family therapy since again a systemic approach suggests that in families people do not simply behave, or feel, or think, but "show" or "communicate" feelings and thoughts to each other through interactive behaviour, over time (see Selvini-Palazzoli *et al.*, 1978). We therefore need to explore change in each of these areas and also across different contexts. For example, it may not be enough to use a Beck Depression Inventory to measure changes in depression in a mother in a family. We also need to observe how or whether the person is able to act, think or feel differently in the presence of others (Jones & Asen, 2000).

As in other psychotherapy outcome studies, the question of change over time and relapse is central. However, systemic practitioners clarify that we would expect fluctuations; for example, that sadness may be intensified according to the unfolding of life-cycle issues. Outcome in family therapy, therefore, offers a more complex and arguably more genuine picture of change, which can be categorized as:

(a) individual;
(b) interactional;
(c) contextual;
(d) time related.

Systemic therapy has, from the outset, made some important distinctions about change, such as distinguishing between first and second order change:

(a) first order—is there more or less of the problem;
(b) second order—reorganization of what the problem means *and* the dynamics around it.

Identifying this emphasis on change of perspective is also echoed in many individual psychotherapies; for example, in cognitive behavioural therapy (CBT) there is a growing awareness that change is not just substituting a dysfunctional belief for a more functional one, but represents an ability to reorganize "core schemas" and fundamental assumptions, which includes an ability to be more reflexive and able to generate novel solutions to solve problems.

The outcome studies

We shall outline some of the findings from the earlier reviews of the efficacy of marital and family therapies, so that we can plot the continuity in findings with the later reviews. Gurman *et al.*, (1986), in their major substantive review, concluded as follows:

(a) the non-behavioural marital and family therapies produce beneficial outcomes in at least two-thirds of cases, and their effects are superior to no treatment;
(b) when both partners/spouses are involved in face-to-face conjoint therapy, there is a greater chance of a positive treatment outcome than when one partner/spouse is treated separately;
(c) the developmental level of the person with the identified psychological problems (for example, child, adolescent, adult) does not affect the treatment outcomes significantly;
(d) the positive effects of both the behavioural and non-behavioural couple and family therapies typically occur in treatments of short duration, for example, one to twenty sessions; and
(e) family therapy is as effective as, and possibly more effective than, many commonly offered (usually individual) treatments for problems attributed to family conflict and relationship difficulties.

During the late 1980s and 1990s, some major meta-analytic reviews of the efficacy of family therapy were published in both American and British journals, such as Hazelrigg *et al.*, (1987); Markus *et al.*, (1990); Shadish *et al.*, (1995); and Goldstein and Miklowitz (1995). The following list of people and problems is found to benefit both clinically and significantly from the marital and family therapies compared with no psychotherapy:

marital/couple distress and conflict;
women with a diagnosis of depression in distressed marriages, treated on an outpatient basis;
adult drinking problems and drug misuse; adolescent substance misuse;
adults with a diagnosis of schizophrenia;

adolescents with a diagnosis of conduct disorder;
young adolescent girls with a diagnosis of anorexia nervosa;
children with a diagnosis of conduct disorder;
aggressive and non-compliant behaviour in children with a diagnosis of Attention Deficit Hyperactive Disorder (ADHD);
children with chronic physical illnesses;
obesity in children;
and cardiovascular risk factors in children.

Importantly, there appears to be no evidence that the couples and family therapies are harmful. No Randomized Control Trial (RCT) study has reported poorer outcomes for treated clients than for untreated control family members (Pinsof & Wynne, 1995).

Alan Carr reviewed the evidence base for practice in family therapy and systemic consultation for the *Journal of Family Therapy*, for child-focused problems (2000a) and adult-focused problems (2000b). He made an interesting departure from the studies reviewed above by including family- and parent-based interventions that drew on cognitive and behavioural models as well as systemic models. He reviewed evidence that supported the effectiveness of family therapy, either as a single treatment intervention or as part of a treatment package. Child-focused referrals for problems such as child abuse and neglect, emotional problems, conduct problems, and psychosomatic problems responded positively to a family-therapy-based intervention (Carr, 2000a). Similarly, his review of adult-focused problems included evidence for the efficacy of a family-based approach for marital distress, mood disorders, anxiety problems, psychotic disorders, drinking problems, chronic pain, and the family management of neurologically impaired adults. Of note in his reviews are the findings that family-based interventions have been applied by a range of mental health professional staff and many of the interventions reviewed are supported by practice manuals.

A more recent example is the successful manual developed by Jones and Asen (2000) for using systemic couple therapy to treat couples where one of the partners is diagnosed with significant depression. Jones and Asen were the research therapists who delivered the systemic therapy as part of the London Depression Intervention Trial (Leff *et al.*, 2000). Such manualized approaches facilitate training, particularly, as in this case, in an area of work that has always been assumed to be less open to therapeutic intervention. The reviews cited above would support the contention that all mental health practitioners could benefit from continuing professional development that included learning and coaching in specific systemic practices that have been found to be helpful. The question remains as to what influences our professional consensus, and whether the RCT studies have an impact on our treatment decisions and conversations with couples and family members about which approaches might best "fit" their preferred styles of thinking and relating.

Despite the relative success of the outcome literature in capturing the effects of the couple and family therapies, there remain a number of knotty methodological and conceptual problems. In fairness, we could say that researching the impact of a group-based intervention will always have problems in determining "whose reality" is being researched and resolving differences in points of view across the family members themselves, the therapists, and observers to the process. Methodological and conceptual problems with the literature include: (a) researching the efficacy of family therapy with a clearer delineation of the severity of the problem; (b) controlling more carefully for attention–placebo effects in the control groups while maintaining a standard of ethical awareness of the costs and impact of participation in control groups; (c) the need for therapist activity to be subject to more process checks; (d) the requirement for more studies to be done that include a larger number of participants; and (e) evaluating outcome across multiple perspectives and multiple levels, for example, first and second order change.

The third generation of outcome researchers, the "progress researchers" (Pinsof & Wynne, 2000), have turned their attention to these problems and have innovated some interesting solutions. They would argue the need for research to link process to outcome, and to ask how family therapy works, but more radically, they would propose that process moments in therapy actually constitute small outcomes. This sets the challenge for the next generation of outcome researchers. Arguably, the empirical base for the evidence-based practice of family therapy is strong and still growing. The "progress researchers" will help develop our thinking about practice-based evidence, and help make the field of outcome research relevant for practitioners through their interest in significant moments of our day to day practice. Many outcome studies and the accumulation of knowledge they offer can be a rather blunt picture. We may end up knowing little about what has really changed and even less about how this has happened. We especially need to know about the latter in order to help us build and shape our therapeutic skills, techniques, and models.

Processes of change in families and family therapy

The family therapy field abounds in theoretical models of the process of change, but less is understood about the active ingredients that promote such changes. Before reviewing some of the work of the family process researchers, we shall summarize again the different approaches to change in the systemic field.

The different schools of thought in the family therapy and systemic field emphasize different levels of change processes in their work, such as change at the level of symptomatic behaviour, change at the level of relationship and family structure, and change at the level of beliefs, held both individually and collectively. For example, the structural school (Minuchin *et al.*, 1996) argues that individuals' felt and lived experiences change when change occurs at the level of family organization and structure. Thus, for example, if a child's parents develop a more unified approach to teamworking and undermine each other's parenting less than before as a result of therapeutic intervention, then the structural approach would expect the child's experience of being parented to change, facilitating other options for the child's behaviour. An example from the schools of the brief and strategic therapies would be based on the understanding that human dilemmas and difficulties can arise from ineffective solutions to problems, maintained because people find themselves unable to generate alternative solutions (Watzlawick *et al.*, 1974). An example from Milan- and post-Milan-based practice would be the use of interventive questioning to identify, highlight, and amplify connections between beliefs, behaviours, and relationships, with change occurring as a result of the development of new perspectives within relationships (Tomm, 1984a,b).

Family psychotherapy process research

The family process researchers have been interested in the processes hypothesized to bring about change in family therapy, a subject of much interest to the practising clinician. Family psychotherapy process research is research that adds to the outcome literature by asking questions about the active ingredients that promote change. Relative to the field of outcome research, there has been less research activity devoted to the study of interpersonal change processes. One of the problems that face researchers is the lack of adequate micro-therapy theory in family therapy. We might presume, then, that psychotherapists and counsellors have resorted to theory and experience as the main source of ideas about how change happens. Interestingly though, many theoretical articles and technique-based workshops tend to focus more on what therapists should do to help bring about change and less on what family members might do. One exception to this is the work of Kuehl and colleagues, who used a process of ethnographic, retrospective interviewing to elucidate accounts of interpersonal change from family members in twelve families who had been through a structural/strategic therapy for help with adolescent substance misuse (Kuehl *et al.*, 1990). Family members identified stages in the therapy process, collectively described as: the introductory meeting; assessment; getting down to basics and generating suggestions; putting suggestions into practice; sharing successes with the counsellor; and troubleshooting and follow-up. Their key findings centred on the connection between reported positive outcomes and family members' perceptions of their counsellor as caring and able, and the connection between dissatisfied clients' perceptions of their counsellor as "on too strict a programme". The flexible use of theory was valued by all respondents. The implications of this process research for the development of the therapeutic relationship centres on their finding that when the therapist is perceived as caring, then family members are more likely to divulge personal information that facilitates *informed* problem-solving. Of particular interest to systemic practitioners was their finding that parents were more prepared to discuss their marital problems in therapy if they had already appreciated that these were upsetting to their children. If not, the therapy stalled at this point if the therapist was too tenacious.

It could be argued that the development of the therapeutic relationship in work with couples, families, and groups is more complex than in work with individuals, and that there are different demands on the therapist's perceptual, conceptual, and executive skills as a result (Tomm & Wright, 1979). Thus, when considering change processes in family and systemic therapy, we need to take account of these differences. For example, the therapist makes interpersonal alliances with each of the family members, some of whom may be in conflict or rivalrous with one another, as well as with the family as a group. Bennun (1989) reminds us that men as fathers find it easier to engage with a family therapist when they feel that their family is liked and viewed positively by the therapist. The emphasis on collaborative relationships makes the potential for "co-therapy" relationships with family members and participation in or observation of family enactments a particularly complex and sensitive process. The therapist has a responsibility to manage the multi-person conversation so all points of view are heard, and the conversation and behavioural exchange does not become destructive.

The thrust of family process research had been the careful observation of behaviours during specified segments of interaction, usually as a form of speech-act analysis. This involved describing behaviours as frequencies or proportions, in an attempt to answer such questions as: (a) what factors might predict early termination of family therapy? (b) what are the common and distinctive features of therapist–client interaction across different modalities of therapy? (c) what is the relationship between participant's gender and aspects of therapy process? (d) what interpersonal changes take place during the course of therapy? The family therapy process researchers were interested to know whether therapy outcome might be predicted or predictable through direct observation of behaviour and comparison of different modes of expressions, rates of participation, and types of response.

Friedlander *et al.*, (1994) reviewed over 30 years' worth of family process research, including naturalistic studies of conjoint therapy in which the focus of the research was the verbal behaviour of the participants during the therapy, or their self-reported perceptions of actual interactions during the therapy. They reviewed thirty-six studies that met their inclusion criteria, dating from 1963. They followed Greenberg's (1986) format for reviewing process in individual psychotherapy, and organized their review on three hierarchical levels of behavioural processes: (a) speech acts during therapy; (b) significant moments of change or incidents during therapy; and (c) the therapeutic relationship.

Speech acts during therapy

Alexander *et al.*, (1976) found that the proportion of defensive to supportive speech acts was significantly higher in families who ended their therapy prematurely. Continuing this theme, Shields *et al.*, (1991) compared families who ended their therapy early with those who ended their therapy in agreement with the therapist. They found that the family groups who ended therapy early were characterized by more in-therapy disagreements with more attempts to structure the therapist, whereas the families who completed therapy engaged in more problem-solving conversations and their therapists were more structuring in response to family disagreements. These findings might suggest that early defensiveness amongst family members, however caused, may predict early termination of therapy. Although we have little further information about the families or their particular contexts, the findings would suggest special attention is given during training to the issues around joining and engagement.

Dowling (1979) reported the first observational study of co-therapy behaviour. She explored the consistency of therapist behaviour across the two different roles of therapist and co-therapist, focusing on five co-therapy pairs. Dowling developed a family therapist behaviour coding scheme, adapted from the Developing Interactive Skills Category System as used by the British Air Transport and Travel Industry Training Board. Audio recordings were sampled from therapy with nine families, from the beginning, middle and ending sessions. She found that therapists behaved similarly with different co-therapists and with different families, supporting the notion that therapists had a consistent co-therapy style. In addition, she used the coding scheme as a self-report device, and found that therapists tended to seek in a co-therapist behaviours they did not exhibit themselves. This lends support to the notion of complementarity of function.

These findings complement those of Hampson and Beavers

(1996). Their study looked at the therapy outcomes for a group of 175 families. They described the families according to the Beavers Systems Model, which differentiates family groups according to their emotional style (on a dimensional scale from close and enmeshed, to balanced, to distancing and disengaged) and their competence (on a dimensional scale from competent and authoritative, to more controlling and authoritarian, to less competent and chaotic). The therapists were asked to rate themselves in terms of "openness/sharing strategy", "power differential", and "partnership with the family" at the third session with each family. They found that those families rated as more competent did well in therapy with those therapists who formed a partnership, disclosed their strategy, and employed a minimal power differential with the family group. However, the families rated as most disturbed, and with a more disengaged emotional style, did better with those therapists who employed a high power differential and lower levels of openness and partnership.

Such findings might well help us begin to understand and explain how the therapy alliance can fail in some instances, and why not all families benefit from therapeutic intervention or the same approach to intervention. Assessment will be helpful in guiding the approach to intervention and expectations about possible outcomes.

Postner *et al.*, (1971) examined family members' verbal behaviours as predictors of outcome. Segments of interaction were analysed at four points in therapy for eleven families. The speech acts were coded broadly into emergency, welfare, or neutral emotional states. Independent judges rated outcomes of the therapy as good or bad. Results from the good outcomes showed that family members tended to speak more to each other during the course of the therapy, made increasingly more welfare statements during the course of the therapy, and that significant changes in emotional expression occurred between the second and sixth sessions.

The findings from the speech act studies reviewed by Friedlander and her colleagues are informative in their own right, but do not add to our accumulated knowledge of *how* change occurs *over time* during successful therapy. In addition, because different investigators have relied on different coding systems within different theoretical frameworks, it is difficult to generalize findings across studies.

Significant moments of change during therapy

The second level of analysis in the studies reviewed by Friedlander *et al.*, (1994) identify significant moments in therapy. Their aim is to elucidate interpersonal change processes through a detailed look at what happens during these "moments", as identified by therapists and family members. An example can be found in the work of Patterson and Forgatch (1985) who identified and coded instances of mothers' non-compliance with the therapist's suggestions. They found that non-compliant responses were more likely to follow therapists' attempts to "teach or confront" mothers, as coded, whereas a decrease in non-compliance was coded following therapists' "support or facilitate" interventions. Using a larger sample from the same child behaviour management project, Patterson and Chamberlain (1988) identified instances of within-session conflict between mothers and fathers. Using path analyses, they suggested that external factors, such as parental stressors, conflict in the marriage, and symptoms of depression, appeared to increase the within-session conflictual behaviour among the family members. This study is important in identifying that external stressors and forces at times may have more of an influence on within-session behaviour, than what happens in the therapy. In addition, they reported high correlations between anti-social behaviour scores for the children, and within-session conflict. They conclude that therapists should attend to the external sources of stress and contextual determinants for family members' behaviour when planning interventions, with the aim of trying to help reduce such parental and marital stress. Although the Patterson studies rely on small samples, they do contain important indicators to the value of systemic thinking and practice.

We shall include here, the work of Charlotte Burck and Stephen Frosh and their colleagues (Burck *et al.*, 1998; Frosh *et al.*, 1996). They make use of a single case approach to develop the use of discourse analysis for the study of change processes at the level of therapy discourse. Although their studies are methodological in orientation, they did find that when a family group and their therapist reported a successful therapy outcome, it was associated with the elaboration of discourses in therapy. For example, if parents held one view of their parenting, which was probably negative, the therapist worked hard to introduce new ways of thinking about their parenting, which may have involved identifying overlooked examples of successes, and so on. It would seem that the ability of the parents to elaborate their own views of their parenting was associated with successful outcome. These small-scale studies conducted by Burck and her colleagues do not allow us to generalize, but do help us understand further the value of established interventions such as, reframing and offering support for what is going well.

The therapeutic relationship

The third level of analysis in the Friedlander *et al.* review is the therapeutic relationship itself. Individual therapists have a long history of exploring the core conditions of therapy, such as therapist warmth, acceptance, empathy, and unconditional regard. The therapeutic alliance is considered to be the vehicle for much psychotherapeutic change. Recent reviews of outcomes in therapy would suggest the therapeutic relationship and client motivation contribute to more of the variance in outcome than does the theoretical orientation of the therapist (Duncan & Miller, 2000). This conclusion connects to the motivational interviewing approaches that explore what the therapist does to increase or decrease clients' motivation to change. Family therapists have not paid as much attention to researching the core ingredients of therapy; rather they have attended more to the strategic and systemic elements of the relationship, such as engaging and joining with the family members, and the development of therapeutic coalitions. In 1978, Gurman and Kniskern concluded, from their review, that the family therapist's ability to establish a positive therapeutic relationship with the family members was most predictive of successful outcome. Since that time very few studies have been published, and only six met the inclusion criteria for the Friedlander *et al.* review reported here.

Shapiro (1974) concluded that greater therapist emotional responsiveness to family members, as measured by questionnaire, predicted client continuance in therapy beyond the initial assessment phase. Family members who were not seen in such a positive light by their therapists tended not to continue in therapy beyond assessment. These ratings were global and did not have other psychometric support. However, they fit the trend of findings reported from other studies. For example, Bennun's (1989) study, mentioned earlier, found not only the importance of perceived therapist liking for the family, but, just as important, the perception that the therapist was competent and structuring of the session.

Pinsof and Catherall (1986) developed a more robust psychometric measure of the therapeutic alliance for family members. They used their measure to explore the development of the therapeutic alliance across family therapy sessions and found that it developed variably rather than uniformly. Their research showed a trend for family members' alliance ratings to be positively correlated with therapists' ratings of outcomes, with most family members rating their therapist positively. Of most interest to us here, perhaps, is their finding that alliances are best understood as multi-dimensional; for example, relating to the therapy tasks, the therapy goals, and the developing therapy bonds; and, as occurring on multiple levels, such as whole system alliances, subsystem alliances, and individual alliances.

Coulahan (1995) provides an interesting account of her six years working as a research therapist in the Maudsley Eating Disorders Trials. She pays special attention to the difficulties involved in trying to engage young people and their families in family therapy and family counselling in order to meet the requirements of a series of outcome studies. One of the key findings from this series of studies was that parents who behaved in more hostile and critical ways towards their adolescent child fared better in the family counselling model, where parents are seen separately from their child (Le Grange *et al.*, 1992). Coulahan writes descriptively about the particular demands on her as a therapist when working this way, and in particular how the therapeutic alliance was strengthened within a model that did not demand working directly with family based conflict and avoided possible power struggles. Follow-up studies found that these families felt less blamed and misunderstood by the therapists (Squire-Dehouck, 1993).

Preliminary conclusions from the process studies

Despite the smaller number of family therapy process studies relative to the outcome studies, Friedlander *et al.* conclude from their review that a few conclusions are possible:

(a) family members' responsiveness to their therapists and their therapists' responsiveness to them appear to be important for successful outcomes;
(b) family members' motivations and commitments to engage in therapeutic activities are predictive of good outcome;
(c) affective changes among family members appear to be crucial for effective therapy;
(d) there are more commonalities among family therapy approaches than differences, with therapists behaving consistently across family work, central in their position with families and skilful in indirect communications; and
(e) individual symptoms as observed in therapy occur in the context of predictable interpersonal events.

We need more research to address how family members themselves construe their experiences in therapy and its effective ingredients. Most of the studies in Friedlander's review relied on observation and self-report through questionnaire. Elliott's (1984) method of Interpersonal Process Recall (IPR), developed within the field of individual psychotherapy, holds promise for the investigation of family members' thinking and reactions during therapy at significant moments, self-identified by family members and therapists. It is a discovery strategy (inductive) developed to examine micro-change processes within therapy sessions, based on the client's ability to be reflexive and give feedback about their experiences. A good example of the use of IPR to exemplify aspects of family therapy experience is found in van Roosmalen's (2001) research. He interviewed parents and children, and himself as the research family therapist, using the IPR methodology of Elliott. He was interested in how best he could work to engage with family members who had a history of experiencing difficulties in interacting with statutory and health services around the needs of the children in the family. Specifically, he used the IPR to look at therapy events that influence the therapeutic alliance. His findings have clear implications for our practice: (a) parents placed importance on how the therapist paid attention in the therapy to the children's communication style and developmental level; (b) the capacity of the therapist to focus and direct the sessions aided a sense of containment and safety for both parents and children; (c) the flexibility of the therapist to collaborate with a family according to the family members, needs was seen as important by all participants; and (d) helping the family members shift from a more individual to a more systemic understanding of the meaning of the problem was seen as helpful to the formation of a strong therapeutic alliance. The challenge for process research is, as ever, in locating behaviour firmly within its social context and avoiding the trap of isolating segments of behaviour from the stream of behaviour.

Asking family members for their feedback

The "user friendly" approaches to systemic practice developed in the UK in response to a number of challenges, including the lack of research attention to family members' experiences in therapy, and to the perceived decline in significance of individual subjectivity within some areas of systemic theorizing.

In 1989, David Howe published a book that put forward some devastating criticisms of family therapy and its practitioners. He interviewed a handful of family members who had received a family therapy service from a group of social workers practising in the UK. The therapy included a mix of strategic and Milan-based approaches, delivered by a single therapist supervised by a team using closed circuit television and an ear-bug. The families interviewed disliked the "hi-tech" approach employed by the team and found it alienating. In particular, they objected to "their" therapist being controlled by some all-seeing, yet unknown team. Howe's critique was helpful in highlighting alienating practices, and it helped mobilize a response that paved the way for more reflecting practices. However, his critique failed to credit a long-standing tradition of debate on the ethics of practice within the family therapy field (for example, Walrond-Skinner & Watson, 1987) and the development of therapy approaches that are both ethically and politically defensible (Waldegrave, 1990).

In direct response to these critiques, Treacher and Carpenter (1983), Reimers and Treacher (1995), and Reimers (2001) have written extensively on the importance of convening and engaging family members in therapy, and of providing them with adequate information in a context that recognizes that many family members find it distressing and problematic to come to therapy. For example, Reimers and Treacher's (1995) series of studies found that family members are often very worried and concerned about what other family members are going to think and say at the first interview. This would suggest that even though family members have known each other for some time, they will need help in "introducing" themselves to each other in the unknown and anxiety-provoking setting of a first family therapy meeting, let alone help with meeting the therapist and any other team members involved in the work! These concerns, along with poor referring practices and any imagined fears of having the children taken away from the family, may go a long way to explaining why some families never arrive for their first appointment or leave therapy in its earliest stages.

Although the relationship of the therapeutic alliance to family therapy effectiveness has not been researched as extensively as in some of the individual psychotherapies, the therapy alliance is held to be a common factor underpinning much effective helping in the family therapies. For example, the research of Bennun (1989), cited earlier, found that fathers were more likely to engage in therapy if they perceived the therapist to be competent, and to show a liking for the family, and to use a problem-solving approach. Mothers, in the same study, preferred the therapist to provide an opportunity for family members to air their common concerns. It is of interest that there was a reported cross-over effect in middle therapy, where mothers preferred a problem-solving approach and fathers came to appreciate "just talking". In a study some ten years later, Campbell (1997) interviewed family members about what they wanted from therapy. He found that they wanted to have their concerns listened to with respect for their efforts to try to solve their problems and they wanted explanations and advice, which they could act on about how to improve their situation.

If we accept the view that engagement is a complex and continuous process throughout the course of therapy (Perlesz *et al.*, 1996), it raises questions about how we review the progress of therapy with our clients, including their direct responses to our therapy practices, such as our use of questions. Reimers (1999) reminds us that some family members have difficulty in dealing with our question–answer process, even when we try to behave in an open and curious way. A participant in Howe's (1989) research described it thus, "Just lots of questions. You answered one and boom! on to the next one. They never got to the bottom of anything".

All of this indicates there is a complex relationship between the processes of convening family members and engaging them in a continuing therapeutic process. User-friendly convening practice, summarized by Reimers (2001) recommends: (a) enabling a smooth referral process, with referrers as well informed about the service as possible; (b) making sure new clients have all the relevant information about the service and the therapy; (c) recognizing that many family members have problems with their literacy—thus not relying too heavily on written information; and (d) offering informal consultation or "talks about talks" in the first meeting—thus giving family members a chance to adjust to new ways of talking to each other and the therapist. Elsewhere in the book (see Chapter Six) we have described the approach to consultation developed by Street *et al.*, (1991), which does not presume that families want therapy. The approach recommended by Reimers assumes therapy has been asked for and agreed to, but still recognizes the novelty and anxiety-provoking nature of the encounter and tries to maximize family members' participation.

The needs and views of children

The needs and views of children in family-oriented services and approaches have received even less research attention. The available research holds a clear message for practitioners: involve the children in the therapy and find ways of engaging them with the use of activities, games, and tasks.

Shalan and Griggs (1998) reviewed UK-generated documentation for children's mental health services and concluded that most of the documentation was paternalistic and not child-centred, leaving them to infer that most children were poorly prepared for therapy.

A few studies have investigated how children participate in family therapy sessions. Some studies have examined how often children speak compared with the adults. For example, Mas *et al.*, (1985) found that children speak far less often than their parents and, when they do speak, tend to express themselves in terms of agreement or disagreement. Cederborg's (1997) study of seven families attending a Swedish child psychiatry clinic used a word space analysis of their videotaped sessions. She found that children produced 3.5% of the words spoken during the meetings, compared with parental output of 56% and therapist output of 37.5%. She described the children's participation as marginal and expressed concern about the impact of this process on children's self esteem, particularly as they may be symptom bearers. Kuehl and colleagues' (1990) ethnographic research of the experiences of adolescent drug users and their parents in family therapy, found that many adolescents did not feel free to speak in front of their parents, and looked for opportunities to foil the therapy between sessions.

Stith *et al.*, (1996) asked children about their experience of therapy and what helped them settle. They found that children appreciated child-centred activities that directly involved them, open discussion of family difficulties that affected them directly, proper explanation of the screen and team, where used, and active participation in the therapy by the therapy team. These findings complement van Roosmalen's study, cited earlier, in which the children said they found it easier to participate in the therapy when the therapist actively involved them with child-centred tasks, a finding also endorsed by the children's parents.

Strickland-Clark and her colleagues (2000) interviewed a small sample of children, aged between eleven and seventeen years, immediately following their family therapy sessions, in order to explore their experiences. The children were invited to recall both helpful and unhelpful events during therapy, using Llewelyn's (1988) approach, and the events were analysed using Comprehensive Process Analysis (Elliott & Shapiro, 1992). The researchers thought the children responded well to the request to give feedback about how their therapy should be managed. The theme of valuing being heard and being included in the therapy was dominant in the feedback. In particular the children spoke about how difficult it was if they thought they were not being listened to or if support for their point of view was not forthcoming, their worries about saying the wrong thing, and how apprehensive they were about coming to therapy if they thought the therapy was designed to reprimand them for bad behaviour. The therapists' attempts to explain how children's views of behaviour might be different to that of their parents, positive reframing of children's behaviour, and a focus on children's strengths rather than weaknesses, seemed especially helpful for this group of children. These findings suggest that more preparation by the therapist to facilitate children's involvement in family therapy is needed.

Children are nearly always brought to therapy by their parents and carers, and if therapy proceeds according to the custom and convenience of adults we risk overlooking their views and potential for contribution. It is questionable to what extent some practitioners understand a child's preferences for communication and their communicative abilities and emotional fluency, and so on. Most of the studies have relied on self-report or analysis of talk time. Little attention, as far as we can see, has focused on children's non-verbal communicative behaviour. This remains an untapped source of hypotheses about children's participation in, and potential to benefit from, the therapy.

The impact of gender and ethnicity on the therapy alliance

The impact of the gender and ethnicity of the therapist on the developing therapy alliance has received little empirical scrutiny despite its prominence in theoretical writings. Gregory and Leslie (1996) report a preliminary survey with sixty-three heterosexual couples. They found that black women clients rated their initial sessions more negatively than white women clients when seeing a white therapist, whereas black men had a more positive reaction than white men to the initial sessions, despite the colour of the therapist. These differences decreased with time. They found no significant effects for the gender of the therapist. These findings support the limited work done so far.

There has been more interest in the effects of gender on therapy process. Of interest here is the variability in the findings, not only because we need to interpret them with caution, but also because such variability is of interest in its own right.

Research into day-to-day conversations between men and

women in Western industrialized societies has focused on patterns of men's dominance, across different aims and types of conversations and conversationalists, across public and private conversations. West and Zimmerman (1977) produced a well-replicated finding that men more frequently interrupt women than do other women. It has been suggested that a woman's role within conversation is to support and maintain the conversation, while men have more control over who speaks and what gets talked about (Fishman, 1983). These findings have informed research interest in what happens in family therapy sessions, while recognizing that as a context for talk it is special because the therapist holds responsibility for making sure some things do get talked about! A therapist may interrupt in a way intended to control the direction of conversation, to facilitate another speaker in having a turn, to introduce a new idea, or to challenge a speaker, among other things. Two studies have investigated the use of interruptions in therapy by both men and women therapists, and these support the notion that both men and women family therapists are inclined to interrupt female clients more often than their male counterparts (Stratford, 1998; Werner-Wilson *et al.*, 1997). Studies that tally the number of interruptions of talk cannot explore the meaning of the interruptions for therapists and for clients. However, they do suggest that we, as therapists, might pay more attention to the importance and role of turn-taking in therapy conversations. It is of interest that the therapists studied expressed surprise when they received feedback about their frequency of interruptions and of their gender bias in interrupting.

Studies that explore the effects of gender on the conversation patterns of supervisors and family therapists in training are even more rare. A study by McHale and Carr (1998) drew on forty episodes of supervision between four matched gender pairs of supervisor and therapist. Their findings ran counter to the gendered findings of the research cited above. They found that the female supervisors in their study used a more directive style, as rated, and was associated with a more resistant trainee style, than for the male supervisors. Thus, they tended to interrupt the trainees more. Conversely, in same gender supervisor–trainee pairs, a collaborative supervisor style was associated equally with either a collaborative or resistant trainee style. Gender had little effect.

Gender effects are complex and interact with a multitude of other variables that may predict better issues of power and status in relationships. However, it could be argued that many women and men who work systemically have developed both directive *and* collaborative skills, perhaps starting from socialization differences in competence. It may be that their training and employment and other selection processes will impact differently on their pre-existing skills and socialized behaviours.

CHAPTER FIVE

Integrative practice: developments in theory

The impact of social constructionism and critical theory

Social constructionists argue that our social world, unlike our physical world is not a pre-given but is actively created. In effect this argument is part of a wider philosophical debate in psychology and the social sciences about whether a positivist version of science can legitimately be applied to the study of human experience and action. Similarly, constructivism had argued that meaning is central and that a psychology that focused predominantly on behaviour was fundamentally limited. However, further to constructivism, social constructionism gives priority to language and argues that language contains the "building blocks", the materials from which we construct our experiences (Foucault, 1975). Like systemic theory, social constructionism also sees interaction and communication as central. Through the processes of conversation, meanings are mutually shaped. Rather than being seen as essentially located within individuals, meanings are seen to be co-constructed, so that with each conversation new meanings, interpretations, and nuances are developed. Importantly, it is suggested that even in our private moments our thinking features internalized conversations with ourselves and with others. I may rehearse conversations that I wish to have with people, or attempt to edit conversations that I have had to get my point across better, and so on.

Social constructionism can be seen to have two distinct strands described as follows.

Top-down—it can be employed to offer a view of human experience as shaped by our internalization of dominant discourses (Hollway, 1989). Not dissimilar in many ways to some ideas expressed in *The Communist Manifesto* (Marx, 1967), this suggests that any society has a range of dominant ideas or ideologies that have power and influence at any particular time. For example, it could be argued that at present the global drug companies have the financial resources and influence to support medical models of various forms of psychological distress because it is in their interest to promote sales of expensive psychiatric medications. Similarly, as will be argued in the next section, the ideas of the dominant gender group, men, have prevailed until recently in most societies in the world.

Bottom-up—in contrast, social constructionism also argues that meanings are shaped locally in everyday conversations. Although we might argue that dominant discourses exist, they are given meanings within the uniqueness of the combinations of specific interactions and the participants' personal biographies. Hence, discourses are not objective entities, but continually shifting waves of meanings. In effect, this can be seen as a more psychological version of social constructionism that emphasizes processes at the micro versus macro level.

Arguably, it is important that both these strands are held in mind. In work with families it may be important to recognize the uniqueness of the meanings that are created but at the same time to recognize that their thinking is also shaped by the cultural context and, in particular, the ideas embedded in our shared language. Again, some of these ideas were elegantly expressed some time ago: "We create reality but not in circumstances of our own choosing" (Marx, 1967, paraphrased).

Also linking these two strands is the notion that meanings are both co-constructed and, importantly, contested and negotiated. This is seen to occur at both the local and the global level. In everyday conversations people are seen to argue over the meanings of their specific actions, but also to contest political and moral discourses, for example over fox-hunting, environmental pollution, or even the value of statistical inference in psychology!

Social constructionism, then, can be seen to contain a number of premises that are closely related to systemic ideas. These are explored below.

There is an emphasis on context and interpersonal processes in creating joint actions. Evidence from other areas, such as developmental psychology (Trevarthen, 1980) suggests that almost from birth babies are connected and synchronise with their mother's actions. Not only does this happen at some reflex or behavioural level but it is shaped by meanings, for example pleasure and comfort. Rapidly mothers and babies develop pre-verbal games, such as teasing, pretending, and so on.

The view that meanings are mutually constructed. Rather than simply or predominantly looking "inside" individuals, social constructionism argues that meanings are jointly constructed and we need to explore the process of interaction when considering the construction of meanings.

Inter-subjectivity. Closely connected to these ideas is the view that for joint action and joint construction of meaning to occur, participants in a social interaction need to be able to develop a mutual view of each other as acting on the basis of meaning. This connects with the "theory of mind", in that we are able to view others as acting intentionally on the basis of views, beliefs, and explanations that may be different from, or similar to, ours. Inter-subjectivity includes participating in shared activities; for example, two friends may discuss a mutual friend to generate a sense of mutual understanding and experience of their recent actions.

Interaction is inevitably strategic. Social constructionism has roots in Wittgenstein's (1951) ideas of language games and in particular the view of pragmatics—the functions that language is employed for and the work that language does. Like early systemic ideas that also drew on this source, in their emphasis on the pragmatics of communication (Watzlawick *et al.*, 1967), social constructionism emphasizes that language use is strategic. For example, it discusses the way that we employ "rhetorical strategies"—ways of using language to achieve certain ends—to persuade, accuse, justify, solicit sympathy or admiration, seduce, and so on. A variety of linguistic strategies is seen to be employed to achieve these ends, such as use of humour, reference to "well known" others, presenting arguments *in extremis*, emphasizing one's honourable intention, use of metaphor and reference to stereotypes or shared images, and stories.

Power is central at both the global level and the level of local interactions. Interactions are seen as inevitably involving a struggle over meanings. Again, this bears resemblance to early strategic ideas that argued that all interactions involve a struggle over power in terms of whose version of events will dominate (Haley, 1969, 1976). Arguably, it is often at the point where people feel unable to persuade by words that they may feel the need to resort to physical means.

Identity is fluid and shifting rather than stable and made up of "personality traits". Perhaps one of the most radical and controversial implications of social constructionism is the challenge to personality theory and more broadly to psychology. It is suggested that identity is fluid and changing rather than fixed and invariant. Likewise, social constructionism argues that the idea of stable beliefs, schemas, and attitudes is flawed (Gergen, 1985; Potter & Wetherell, 1987). This is a direct challenge to many psychological approaches, such as cognitive behavioural therapies, which attempt to alter patterns of "dysfunctional" beliefs.

Social constructionism has offered some influential new perspectives for family therapy, as it has for psychology and social sciences more generally. The influence has been both at a broader conceptual level and in terms of some specific approaches in the practice of family therapy. It has alerted therapists to consider the broader social contexts, such as the dominant ideas that shape the behaviour end beliefs of family members. This includes a consideration of how, for example, medical ideas of "mental illness" may pervade and impede their thinking, gender expectation, and ideas about "strength" and "weakness" in family members. The ideas contribute to the cycles of blame, accusation, and sense of failure that families may experience. Related to this, social constructionism alerts us as professionals to examine the bases of our own beliefs, ideologies, and prejudices derived from our professional and private contexts.

More specifically, it has prompted a move for family therapy to become less expert and to work collaboratively with families in creating new meanings rather than to attempt to direct or guide therapy. One of the most striking examples of this movement has been the development of reflecting teams, discussed later in this chapter.

The feminist critiques and working with difference

The emphasis on culture and ideology or discourse separates social constructionism from constructivism. In effect, although interactions are central, they are seen as also shaped by common ideology and discourse—sets of interconnected beliefs held in common in any given culture. Early social constructionism, however, could be seen as pluralistic in that society was viewed as a range of competing or contested discourses. However, fuelled by input from feminist theories, which in turn were based in Marxist analysis, social constructionists have argued (Foucault, 1975; White & Epston, 1990) that the discourses that are available in a given culture at any time are intimately linked to structures of power. As an example, until recently men have had the power to define what were acceptable female identities; women could not vote, were supposed to stay at home with their children, were not expected to enter professions, or to be sexually aggressive. Similarly, inequalities between races have been maintained by structural power that, in turn, can shape and combine with ideological power. Such an analysis represents some stark contrasts to constructivism. Rather than seeing people as inevitably free to construe the world in their personal and subjective ways, social constructionism proposes that in any given culture there are common materials, building blocks from which identities and relationships are constructed. Further, it maintains that some members of our society have more power than others to design and construct identities; for example, the medical profession has the power to assign a variety of labels, such as "schizophrenic" or "anorexic", to people. In turn, members of the medical professions are required to act in certain ways as part of their position in the social order; they are not simply free to do otherwise.

Williams and Watson (1994) argued in an edition of *Clinical Psychology Forum* that clinical psychologists have been slower than some other professional groups, such as social workers, in identifying links between social inequalities and psychological distress. They went on to say that by ignoring these links we serve, albeit inadvertently, the interests of privileged social groups. They recognized that, typically, people come into clinical psychology to serve their fellow humans, not to support unjust social divisions. Part of their solution to this dilemma lay in acknowledging sexual and other inequalities in psychological distress, in developing a knowledge base by talking to women users and ex-users of our mental health services, in reading theory and research on women and men and mental health, and in being mindful of their own experiences of power and powerlessness.

In this section we shall focus on gender and gender stereotyping, and the links between feminist theorizing and systemic practices when working with household family groups.

Feminist thinking has highlighted (a) that men's experience in the world has been more widely articulated than that of women; (b) that men and women are likely to have different experiences of self as a result of differences in socialization practices; (c) that women do not have equality of opportunity as yet, despite recent legislation throughout much of Europe; and (e) has placed the family in historical context and challenged views of family life as given. These critiques have given rise to calls to re-examine family theories and family life, including women's and men's rights and responsibilities, and, in particular, to re-examine theories and practices informing family systems practices (Burck & Speed, 1995). Earlier family therapy thinking and practice was specifically criticized for assuming that men and women had equality of opportunity, both within and outside the home (Hare Mustin, 1986). The rise of gender-sensitive practice was in direct response to these calls for a re-examination of social roles and family therapists' reflexive position as users of theory who were subject to the same processes of acculturation as the people they served.

Gender has been defined as a social construct which assigns certain qualities and social roles to one sex, and others to the other sex, thus defining what is commonly considered masculine or feminine at certain times and places. Conversely, gender stereotyping has been defined as regarding certain behaviours and attributes as appropriate to only one sex, and then behaving as if these differences are natural rather than socially constructed (Williams & Watson, 1988). Penfold and Walker (1984) outlined two sets of processes that could be said to maintain inequality between social groups: those that obscure the existence of inequality, and those which make it hard to react against inequality. With respect to gender inequality, ideologies that justify the existence of inequality by calling it "natural" or "morally correct"; ideologies which ignore violent means of controlling women by calling it "deserved"; ideologies which justify inequality by calling it "complementary"; and ideologies which encourage women to look inside themselves for the source of their distress rather than to their social position, are examples of the former processes. Processes which make it hard to react against inequality include: women's larger economic dependency on men; women's reliance on part-time, less well paid jobs; women's continued restricted access to the social institutions that make laws and create wealth; and personal risks to women of challenging the status quo.

Systemically speaking, power has been defined in a number of ways that challenge our practice as psychotherapists. For example, power is being in a position to block feedback; or lies in being able to define reality and have other people accept that definition; or is thought to be relative to our access to resources or centres of influence.

Interpersonal power bases have been defined by Williams and Watson (1988). They argue that men and women have differential access to power bases organized by their gender. Men are said to rely on economic power, ascribed power, physical strength, contractual power, informational power, and gendered language use. Women are said to rely on relational and affective power, domestic, reproductive, and sexual power bases. Part of the value in deconstructing the resources available to ourselves and our clients, such as the allocation of resources and privileged access to those resources, lies in beginning to talk about what people sometimes feel they cannot talk about or do not know how to talk about. The experience of poverty, for example, may have an indirect effect on a person's view of themselves and others, and may be an important contextual determinant of behaviour, yet may not ever be spoken about directly in the therapy setting. Acknowledging our own position in the system, as members of a middle-class professional grouping with power to define clients' reality and to privilege some information over others, or as providers of court-mandated therapeutic work, for example, can be the first step towards addressing the constraints on all participants and asking whether it is possible still to have an interesting conversation.

Thinking about the relationship between power and powerlessness in our work challenges us to explore how abuses of power, such as violent behaviour, can occur as a result of feeling powerless, or how believing that one's own actions have no effect could be harmful to others when operating within these premises. Differentiating between personal power and structural power, i.e. what an individual can do and what needs to happen at an organizational level, and in that, acknowledging the limits of our own power and influence, are important considerations in our work with clients, families, and their relationships with larger groups and social institutions. Supervision can help address our own responses to feeling powerless in therapy. For example, getting into an argument you cannot win with one or more family members, when working on your own, seems a common experience among people we have supervised over the years.

The issue of power in therapy is many-layered. At times we may perceive, or even feel indignant about, "destructive" discourses that are shaping the actions and experiences in a family. However, we have to be careful in our "recognition" of inequalities that we do not in turn impose our value system on a family. For instance, we may feel that a woman is being trapped in traditional roles of passivity and dependence in a relationship. Yet we have worked with couples where the woman has said "I am not a feminist, I still want my husband to take the lead in situations such as initiating sexual intimacy." In such situations we may need to be careful to invite families to explore issues of power and gender without incidentally imposing our values and, in fact, a similar process of oppression on them. Genograms can be used in a potentially non-oppressive way for exploring with families the discourses of power and gender.

An analysis of power and discourse reminds us that dominant

ideas and beliefs in any given culture shape not only the patterns and nature of relationships between people but also our private inner worlds. Possibly it is at our most private moments, physically alone, deep in thought that, we are most likely to be caught in the currents of dominant discourses. For example, when we talk to ourselves in terms such as: "I should have been more in control", "I ought to have been more honest" or "Why am I so disorganized?", this is when we are immersed in dominant ideas about what it is to be "healthy, normal, and functional".

Gender-sensitive approaches to systemic practice are not embodied as a set of skills or techniques. Gender sensitivity is more a process that is negotiated between the therapist and the family members when exploring opportunities to negotiate members' needs and the tensions between individual and group needs. This is based on the view that therapy is political; that it concerns the allocation and distribution of resources. There are a number of factors that are thought to play a part in such a process. They will be discussed in turn.

If we accept the reflexive position that we are part of the system under observation, subject to the same influences of cultural and gender role expectations and stereotyping, and arguably occupying a powerful position as members of a professional grouping, we then have an ethical obligation to examine how these processes impact on relationships between family members, between family members and social institutions, and between family members and ourselves, including the social institutions we represent. Such a process of examination during the therapy emphasizes the social context as an important systemic determinant of behaviour and, further, recognizes that men and women encounter some unique problems as a result of their different socialization experiences.

Examining our own prejudices and values regarding gender and power as they are expressed in therapy and supervision, and how they might dovetail with theoretical prescriptiveness, can help maintain a lightness of approach. We have discussed earlier the concern that family life-cycle models can privilege certain experiences and choices over others. Broadening our conceptualizations to explore a range of life-style choices can release us from discussions of family life in terms of stereotypic roles. Supervision can provide a forum for looking at how much we use our gendered selves in therapy, both deliberately and unselfconsciously. We have the potential to challenge and model alternatives to gender stereotypes; for example, both men and women therapists may show competence and be active in therapy, while offering empathy, respect, and careful listening. Not surprisingly, some couple therapists choose to work in mixed co-therapy pairs for the opportunities afforded to model different styles of communication and negotiation between men and women.

As practitioners, we can ask questions that make explicit some of the issues, choices, decisions, and behaviours that show to what extent reciprocity and equality exist between men and women in the family. The following questions are examples of those we might ask of a couple.

> How did you decide who would work outside the home, and who would work inside the home, looking after the children?
> How much flexibility do you think you have or want in these arrangements?
> How satisfied are you with these arrangements?
> Who benefits most and who carries most cost?
> Are there differences in your roles inside and outside the family?

The assumption is that the allocation of roles and tasks solely on the basis of gender is to be minimized. If, then, we facilitate consideration of a wider range of perspectives and solutions, we need to pay attention to the implications for both partners. For example, if discussing parental teamwork and shared responsibilities, we need to check that the woman is willing to share parental responsibility, and has other ways of expressing her competence, and that the man is willing to bear the cost in the workplace of becoming more involved with his family.

Positive reframing and relabelling can be used to shift conceptual and emotional perspectives; for example, reinterpreting what might be seen as personal inadequacy as socially prescribed. This can be achieved by exploring with men and women what they have been taught about theirs and each others' social roles, in comparison to their actual competencies, interests and needs. A genogram is a useful tool for exploring the inter-generational transmission of ideas and beliefs about men and women in the family.

Williams and Watson's (1988) analysis of interpersonal power bases is helpful in formulating questions about how the presence or withdrawal of these sources of power affect everyday family processes, such as decision-making, conflict resolution, and negotiation.

Much less has been written about men in relation to gender sensitivity. It is helpful to draw out men's experiences and the costs and benefits to them of certain life-style choices, for example, pursuing a gendered career path. O'Brien (1990) has reviewed research which suggests that men are less likely than women to seek help about emotional concerns, and that when they do seek help and take restorative action, it is much later on in the process. Bennun (1989) suggests that men are harder to convene in couples and family work, and cites a number of reasons, including men's responsibilities in the workplace clashing with the timing of clinic appointments, or accepting the normative assumption that the mother takes responsibility for child care and dealing with the professional workers. A small-scale research study by Walters *et al.*, (2001) challenged the idea that work hours and family roles may not be as important predictors of fathers' attendance at family therapy meetings as their relationships with their own fathers and their current relationships with their own partners. So, if fathers reported more positive experiences with their own fathers and more satisfying relationships with their own partners, they were more likely to attend clinic appointments. The implication for our practice is that we should proactively attempt to engage fathers whose attendance is poor, and given the finding of the importance of couple relationship satisfaction, perhaps not to too readily rely on the partner to convene a father without trying to speak to him as well.

It is our view that we should take seriously the implications for men and women in families of not successfully engaging men in therapeutic work with their families. Bennun suggests that men are more likely to return for a second appointment if they think the therapist has shown a liking for their family, is competent, has structured the first session, and has a problem-solving approach. Walters *et al.*, (2001) suggest we should be sure to positively connote fathers' roles in families. Interestingly, a few meetings into the therapy, men are reported to enjoy "just talking". This would suggest that one dilemma that needs careful thought is how to help men manage their vulnerability in a therapy meeting, and then help them to shift back home, as it were, taking the vulnerability back into their life. The challenge for the therapist is to help men reflect on their experiences and how their lives are storied within normative and prevailing views of masculinity, especially beliefs about what can be said publicly about their inner commentary, such as, inner thoughts and private fears and hopes.

Asking men what they think the impact of their behaviour is on family members, how they came to be like this, what are the advantages and disadvantages for the man of his behaviour, is one way to open a conversation that challenges prevailing views. However, the therapist must avoid being perceived as persecutory. In our experience, men sometimes accuse their female partners of trying to make them like women, so the danger for the woman therapist is of being seen to ask the same things of him as his female partner. If a man is uncomfortable with expertise in a woman therapist, and becomes competitive, or needs always to know and be certain, the woman therapist (or the man therapist in a similar situation) needs to prevent a symmetrical escalation and not take on responsibility for the man in the ways women traditionally have. In our view these are pertinent issues for supervision, and dilemmas such as these probably go some way towards understanding the preference for some therapists to work in mixed sex co-therapy pairs, where issues of transference and counter-transference can more easily be addressed.

Working with cultural difference

Like other forms of therapy, family therapy is confronted with a complex task in relation to cultural differences. There may well be multi-faceted problems and challenges that confront different ethnic groupings within particular localities. Practitioners and researchers need to address these issues directly. Perhaps for psychologists and other social scientists there are particular tensions. For example, one of the traditions in psychology has been to map commonalities; to study what aspects of human actions and experiences are universal. Psychology abounds with examples: the Piagetian stages, individual differences, psychodynamic views of development, models of cognitive processes, attachment patterns, and so on. One of us, AV, would want to argue that much of the early search for commonality between men's and women's abilities was in part a response to perceived inequality; i.e. in terms of abilities, there were no empirical reasons why women could not take advantage of higher education, and work in professions and occupations claimed as a male preserve. The discipline of psychology held the potential to undermine any claims that women were not suited for certain kinds of activity and employment. However, the field was fraught with contradictions. For example, only relatively recently has it been pointed out (Gilligan, 1982) that the general findings supposedly established in the majority of psychological research were based on studies of boys and men and excluded women and girls. Where females were included, differences between the genders were often ignored in the service of statistical techniques based upon averaged scores.

Such criticisms have been levelled at research and practice that make assumptions about white homogeneity (Turner, 2001). It could be said the search for commonality went too far, in that it obscured the differences in resources and sources of influence between men and women, boys and girls. Given this emphasis on commonality, it was tempting also to marginalize the influence of cultural differences. Yet to do so has been shown to be dangerous, especially in clinical practice. A powerful and well-reported example has been the tendency to over-diagnose acute forms of distress, such as schizophrenia in Afro-Caribbean populations in the UK (Fernando, 1991). The dangers and issues are multi-layered. For example, we may use culture as a map in our clinical practice, but unless we can find ways to be sensitive to intra-group differences, we risk making generalizations that only serve to reinforce unhelpful stereotypes. For us, the tension lies both in acknowledging that we all may want to be seen as part of a larger human group and in paying attention to differences that may well be self-defining.

Culture is often described as systems of shared beliefs, meanings, values, and practices (Foucault, 1980; Gergen, 1982). These norms and customs will be situated within, and mutually influenced by, different contexts, social, historical, economic, and so on. Thus, culture is often thought to be an active and living process that is created and re-created. This view of culture as process is fundamental to the social constructionist view of the creation of social realities, whereby interactions between people allow them to see and understand events, actions, and objects in particular ways. Thus, the signifying practices of a culture at any given time could be observed and explored in patterns of interaction between people, their use of language, and the images and themes they draw on and create, within their day-to-day routines of living together. Ethnicity, as a term, often refers to a collectivity or community that shares common attributes to do with cultural practices and shared history (Phoenix, 2001). This definition of ethnicity applies to everyone, as everyone can be said to have an ethnicity. We recognize that the terminology around culture and ethnicity changes often and is subject to hot debate, probably because the terms carry understandings that have sociopolitical consequences for people's lives.

The implications are profound for clinical practice of a reflexive position that acknowledges one's own ethnicity *and* moral position in some of the debates around terminology and labelling (D'Ardenne & Mahtani, 1999). Regular consultation and supervision of our thinking and practice keeps alive our ability to manage these tensions in our work. Similar distinctions to those drawn in the field of gender-sensitive practice have been made between cultural awareness and culturally sensitive practices, highlighting the role of training in promoting sensitive practice. For example, many writers and trainers in the systemic field have developed the *cultural* genogram as both a clinical and a training tool (Halevy, 1998; Hardy & Laszloffy, 1995). As a reflexive training tool, it is based on the belief that in order to practice ethically, systemic practitioners need to understand themselves, how they see others and to think about how these issues are located in cultural contexts. Importantly, Foucault (1980)—and Marx before him—argued that dominant ideas, discourses and ideologies are often most powerful and pernicious when they are "invisible", i.e. when they are "taken for granted" truths, "self-evident" or regarded as "common sense". The cultural genogram has been shown to be particularly sensitive when used to explore contradictions held within the notion of culture as a fluid concept, particularly as we may be inclined to hold on to cultural norms. Additionally, the genogram is also a useful vehicle for the exploration of ethnicity, particularly the less visible forms of white ethnicity, as the process of constructing the genogram pays such close attention to the transmission of intergenerational beliefs and practices.

When preparing a cultural genogram, Hardy and Laszloffy (1995) recommend we define our culture of origin and identify intercultural marriages and partnerships, using colours to denote differences. The next step involves identifying some key organizing principles of our sense of ethnicity, such as issues of pride and shame, and using symbols for their representation. They suggest asking specific questions to stimulate discussion around possible organizing principles, such as: what is the importance of geography, regionality, social class, employment, and religion within the extended family, and how are they valued? Are there patterns of migration and experiences of oppression? How does the extended family view outsiders and insiders to the group, especially where some cultural differences have been identified? How does the group deal with sources of conflict?

Exploring the relevance of this cultural exploration for our clinical practice is the last step in the process and possibly the most challenging. We are asked to consider what aspects of our culture of origin we have most ease in owning, and most difficulty in owning, while considering the implications for the ease or difficulty in our work with different groups of people.

Links to cognitive approaches

Personal construct theory

Personal construct theory was developed by George Kelly (1955) and can be seen as part of a humanistic movement in psychology that emphasized personal choice. Its philosophical roots were in phenomenology and especially in Kant's (1791) view that reality was subjective—we could only ever know the world through our personal lenses. This view of the world as subjective and an active construction also underpins the movement in the second phase of Family Therapy. In addition, Kelly proposed that our views and our actions are systemically related: our constructs shape our actions and the effects of our actions in turn shape our constructs. He proposed a metaphor of "Man the Scientist", as people continually engaged in the process of developing and testing their views of the world. Kelly offered a comprehensive theory that argued that our beliefs or constructs were organized hierarchically so that superordinate constructs or core beliefs shaped the other, more specific, ones. Further, he proposed that our constructs were essentially bipolar—they were based on the identification of difference. The meaning of an action was given in contrast to its opposite. For example, if I see someone as honourable this is in contrast to a view of being dishonourable or corrupt. This notion of contrast was also central to systems theory, which likewise suggested that a system operated *as if*, following a rule premised on a calibration in terms of what is acceptable versus non-acceptable in families and other systems. In a family there may be a concern that its members were too emotionally distant from each other as opposed to emotionally over-involved.

Specifically, personal construct theory (PCT), has been developed in the context of family therapy by Harry Procter (1985). He incorporated Kelly's ideas into a, family construct psychology (FCP), which employed two further core ideas:

- *Sociality*—in order to have a relationship people need to develop ideas about each other's ideas, views of each other's inner worlds or constructs,
- *Commonality*—people also hold beliefs in common with each other, and share ways of seeing events.

In relation to family therapy, Procter (1981) suggested that the dynamics in families become organized around constructs or bipolar division. Furthermore, family members have come to share these constructions even though they may contest them, which in turn shapes their interactional processes, which then shape and support their beliefs. For example, in a family with a clinical problem a shared belief typically develops that the problem predominantly resides in one of them. A young teenage girl may exhibit anorexia, in contrast to the others who do not have this problem. This may imply that she is "ill" or "abnormal" whereas they are "normal" and "healthy". Increasingly, their dynamics may become organized around this bipolarity, leading to exasperated efforts to "get her better", in which case their problems will dissolve.

FCP offers an elegant way of describing the development and

maintenance of problems in a family by revealing how these beliefs may become increasingly polarized and rigid or "pre-emptive" over time. As with CBT, the direction of therapy suggested is to work with families to move towards less rigid and more "propositional" construings—to contemplate that there may be alternative ways of seeing their situation. In therapy the process may consist of invitations to family members to experiment with employing different ways of construing the situation. Central to this is to employ a further aspect of Kelly's theory, which emphasizes that progress and change occur through processes of validation. He argued that threats of invalidation of our constructs produce strong emotional reactions of fear, anxiety, and hostility, which block change and result in hardening of our thinking. This link between thinking and "negative" emotions has also been proposed in cognitive approaches. Therapy, therefore, invites families to contemplate positive and validating constructions of their situations as a step towards change. As with other therapies, there is a fine balance to be found here between such attempts to reframe a family's situation and clearly listening to, and accepting the legitimacy of, their own construings. Kelly saw therapy as similar to the relationship between a researcher and her supervisor. The supervisor assists the researcher in her experiments and investigations, and together they consider and develop different interpretations of the data resulting from the researcher's investigations.

Cognitive behaviour therapy influences

Behaviour therapists and cognitive behaviour therapists are interested increasingly in the utility of family systems ideas and practices. Emmelkamp and Foa (1983) have written about three sources of treatment failure in CBT, one of which is the neglect of, and/or the incomplete assessment of, the social contingencies and factors affecting clients' problems; in particular, the extent to which any client's behaviour is embedded in long-standing and habitual patterns of family interaction, expectations, and beliefs. The realization that some treatment failures might result from an incomplete assessment of powerful social contingencies has led some cognitive therapists to ask what additional help their clients might need in order to benefit fully from their therapies.

Bandura and Goldman (1995) describe how they developed a family systems and cognitive behavioural analysis for use during assessment to address the above issues. They acknowledge that family systems, models and cognitive behavioural models have different theoretical underpinnings, and do not attempt any theoretical integration. Rather, they point to the areas of overlap and how these can be useful in practice, such as the joint emphasis on beliefs and rule systems governing behaviour; the importance of attributions and expectations in perceptions of self and others, and the recognition of options for change; the emphasis on problem-solving patterns; and the significance of interpersonal contingencies to the understanding of symptomatic behaviour. Thus, in therapy, the focus on training in cognitive and behavioural skills to improve and enhance adaptive coping can involve the modification of social and other environmental contingencies that influence clients' problems.

This is an interesting and useful area of overlap, Bandura and Goldman would argue, because the family systems' approaches also focus on identifying and interrupting interactional sequences that are thought to influence symptomatic behaviour. Some of these interactional sequences are thought not to be reducible to the level of individual behaviour as they are unique to systems functioning. Examples might include communication processes, issues of power and hierarchical organization in relationships, and patterns of relational disengagement and over-involvement. Family systems' ideas can help cognitive therapists expand their functional analyses to include extended interactional analyses underpinned by circular models of causality, rather than the linear models of reinforcement contingencies. Systemic analyses and practices can be used to help understand and overcome difficulties experienced by clients during the therapeutic change process, such as the broader social and relational costs associated with change, the clients' involvement in family-wide dilemmas, and the influence of past and present family processes on the content and function of cognitive schemata.

The conceptual shift to a focus on narrative

> What ... is the nature of the therapeutic task? It is for the family to discover that their experience can be witnessed and respected, that

> they can be recognised and not isolated, that it is possible to be touched by this vicious piece of the "real" and come back without going mad. [Frosh, 1997]

Recent years have seen a growing interest in ideas of narrative and their relevance to our work as psychotherapists. Arguably most of the psychotherapies work in the narrative tradition *de facto*, so here we shall discuss some of the methods associated with the work of White and Epston (1990), which overlap with cognitive behavioural methods such as the use of "externalization" and "unique outcomes" in therapeutic work.

The backdrop to the use of these techniques is an assumption shared by all disciplines interested in the development of meaning in human interaction, that people tell stories or narratives about themselves and others, which can be understood as individual or collective constructions of experience with a history, a present, and a future. It is assumed that meanings ascribed to the history give meanings to the present and offer possibilities for the future. The articulation and juxtaposition of meaning across time in a therapeutic context is considered by many psychotherapy approaches to provide a hinge on which changes in meaning can be explored. The focus for narrative practice is the core belief in people's potential for change and a recognition of the profound effects of conversation, language and stories on therapist and client (O'Hanlon, 1994). Many narrative-informed therapists work with individuals, and share fundamental premises with other individually oriented therapies such as, holding as central the connections between the person, their emotional experience, and the therapist. Narrative-informed therapists take this premise further than some psychodynamically informed therapists by their reflexive stance, so that the client's lived experience is believed to be not only the client's story, but also the lived experience of the client and therapist working together.

Narrative approaches emphasize that our beliefs and understandings are fundamentally structured into stories or narratives that connect events, experiences, actions, and feelings over time. Although sharing some of the same territory, a narrative is essentially diachronic versus synchronic. Cognitive approaches and, arguably, PCT to some extent tend to place the emphasis on the contemporary nature of construings rather than as extended over time. A central aspect of narrative approaches is that our sense of identity consists of a set of stories or narratives about past events, current events, and our potential futures. In addition, a central division here is between our preferred or desired view of self and an actual or, in some cases, non-preferred or deviant view. This sense of preferred versus non-preferred stories also connects to our socially shared world or reality. The writer Salman Rushdie uses a metaphor of a "sea of stories" to describe the idea that in any given culture there is a repertoire of shared stories—from *Sleeping Beauty* to the Prodigal Son. Some of these have been written in formal terms, others in a more informal way from the currency of ideas—the struggle against adversity of the plucky underdog, and so on. In addition, there are personal stories that develop within families. Narrative therapy emphasizes how these stories have a place in culture and transmit a continuity of ideas over time. In families they give a map to our experiences and relationships with each other. This feature of narratives as both personal and culturally shared, prompts narrative therapists to work in and reflect on both spheres and in the spaces connecting private and public experience.

For narrative therapists, language is central and within language the phrases, metaphors, and proverbs construct a continuity of ideas. In effect, it is through language that a cultural evolution takes place. Narrative therapy is then centrally concerned with the stories that people hold about themselves and each other. In turn, it seeks to reveal or discover with families how particular stories may be holding them in positions of distress. Of particular significance here are stories about deficit and essential personality characteristics. These also connect with medical models that feature stories of illness and abnormality. A core idea shaping narrative therapies is to expose these negative stories and explore how they are serving to maintain problems. One "technique" frequently employed is to "externalize" the problems by looking, for example, at how "anorexia" has come to dominate and terrorize life in a family. Externalizing the problem is fundamentally about revealing the operation of oppressive stories about anorexia as a form of failure, manipulation, attack on the mother, and so on. In addition, alternative stories may be explored; for example, how anorexia might be promoted by a culture that emphasizes the need to control women's bodies and gives undue importance to women in terms of their appearance.

The narrative approach to exploring people's stories in therapy can be made systemic (a) by exploring the connections between the beliefs and stories from everyone involved about an event of import; (b) by generating multi-perspectives about these events; and (c) by exploring the fit between older and more current stories or accounts about self, others, events, and the connections between them. We can maintain our systemic focus when moving beyond these therapeutic explorations towards the construction of preferred stories, by (a) exploring people's preferred ideas about events; (b) sharing our professional knowledge in the service of these good ideas; (c) reflecting further on the fit between different ideas; (d) addressing the psychological and relational implications and consequences of these different ideas on people and their relationships; and (e) exploring the implications for action (Fredman, 1997).

White and Epston (1990) have summarized some of the key elements of a narrative approach to therapeutic practice which, when used in combination, give the approach its distinctive narrative flavour. We list these elements, as they show areas of helpful overlap with systemic and cognitive therapies and clinical psychology practice as currently taught:

- exploring relevant aspects of lived experience and developing varying perspectives on this;
- exploring the connectedness of events and relationships over time;
- exploring implicit meanings with exploratory conversation;
- identifying those influences which affect the "ownership/authorship" of stories and emphasizing the person as a participant in the story with some power to re-author it;
- identifying dominant and subjugated discourses in a person's accounts and the prevailing arrangements of privilege and power;
- using different "languages" to describe experience and construct new stories;
- mapping the influence of the problem on a person's life and relationships;
- establishing conditions in which the subject of the story becomes the privileged author;

- externalizing the problem;
- recognizing unique outcomes.

The method of externalizing has much in common with cognitive behavioural therapies and gestalt work. It encourages people to objectify, and sometimes personify, difficult problems. This way, the problem becomes external to the person and capable of being described, addressed, talked about, and so on. Thus, if fixed or inherent qualities have been attributed to the person, those same qualities become more fluid and dynamic in this process, just as they might using other systemic techniques such as circular questioning. At the same time, family members trying to help solve the problem may have become dispirited by the apparent lack of success, and subjected themselves to a similar process of self-reinforcing negative attribution. The effects of this process can be heard when family members come to their first meeting. They are likely to describe themselves and their difficulties using a "problem-saturated description" and this becomes the "dominant story of family life" (White, 1989). Thus, the process of externalization helps all family members separate themselves and their relationships from the problem, and opens up opportunities for them to begin to describe themselves and their efforts anew, using systemic processes of reframing and positive connotation.

Externalizing the problem has similar effects to that of Socratic questioning, used by cognitive therapists, whereby some psychological distance is created in relation to a problem that felt overwhelming, or that overwhelmed a person's ability to think *about* it. Similarly, gestalt therapists might personify some aspects of a person's problem. For example, a child who has recurrent stomach-aches with no apparent organic cause, and who is struggling to attend school, might be asked to talk to her stomach-ache, which might be named and "invited" to sit in the adjacent chair, so to speak. Such a procedure would hope to help the child articulate the basis of her worries and concerns.

Another version of a narrative approach has been developed by Eron and Lund (1993) that is closely connected with FCP developed by Procter (1985), in terms of offering a way of connecting cycles of actions and beliefs. However, instead of a focus on constructs, Eron and Lund speak instead of the preferred and non-preferred narratives that family members hold. The schisms or disjunctions between our preferred and non-preferred stories is seen as central. For example, we may feel sad, angry, depressed or desperate when we feel there is a strong split between the two. Eron and Lund illustrate this by describing how a story of depressions may evolve in a family where Al—the father—is recovering from having suffered a heart attack (Figure 1).

They describe how the cycle of narratives and actions based on them can lead to an escalation of the problems. As the cycle progresses Al comes to see himself as less and less capable, and the family members come to see themselves as incapable. The family also come to see Al as ungrateful and he, in turn, comes to resent them and sees them as interfering and disrespectful. In this cycle we can see dominant, culturally-shared stories about what it is to be a man and a father, what it is to be children, the structure of family life, and the impacts of illness, as well as the presence of trans-generational family stories. In this case, there was a story that Al's father had, in his later years, become chronically depressed, alcoholic, and a liability on his family. This spectre of dependency haunted Al and the family.

Eron and Lund's form of narrative therapy involves working with the family to consider both alternative stories and experimenting with alternative ways of acting, i.e. attempted solutions. As an example, discussions take place about the differences between Al and his father, about times that Al had been competent and what he can still do, and how his strength may be slowly regained. Also, a story of how important it is in convalescence to stay active and to exercise is considered, so that the family works together to enable Al

	Al (the father)	**Family members**
Viewing	Prefers to see himself as the capable caretaker of his family, but this view is shaken. He wonders: Will family members still see me as capable? Will I wind up like my father?	Prefer to see themselves as helpful. They notice that Al is acting despondent and hope to lift his spirits.
Doing	After the onset of his illness, acts despondent	Act "helpful" to try to cheer Al up

Figure 1. The effect of a schism between the preferred and non-preferred stories within a family when the father is ill.

progressively to do more. Eron and Lund's approach bears resemblance to the solution-focused approaches discussed earlier, and draws heavily on systemic notions of circularity and feedback.

The narrative approach has certain limitations for some areas of our practice as psychotherapists. Its over-reliance on narrative risks excluding those people who find the articulation of their experiences more difficult, or whose ability to articulate is constrained by some form of disability. Further, the approach privileges what is said, rather than the way in which it is said, and de-emphasizes the role of observation and the importance of non-verbal communication in therapy and in people's lives. There is a risk that the emphasis on authorship of one's own stories plays down the role of social, political, and economic factors on people's lived experience, despite the recognition within the approach of the influence of power arrangements. This is a similar trap for many approaches to individual practice, not just narrative-informed ones, and is why we would suggest holding a systemic frame at all times. This keeps us mindful of connections—between people, events, and history and between the wider structural arrangements of power and resources. Clearly, assessment is important to help judge the fit between your approach and your clients' style and their preferences for working and your shared formulation and goals. The narrative approaches offer interesting and creative possibilities for the negotiation of change. Their relative newness in the psychotherapy field means that they have not been subjected to the rigorous scrutiny of outcome research. However, we would suggest there is much of value in the narrative approaches, drawing as they do on aspects of well established good practice within other models of psychotherapy.

Reflecting processes and reflexive practice

The use of reflecting processes within the practice of systemic psychotherapists has an interesting, thoughtful, and long history. We shall highlight some contributions that in our view have harnessed the therapeutic potential of multiple observers and perspectives in ways that can be consonant with common mental health practice.

Kingston and Smith (1983) developed an approach to in-room

consultation at a time when preferred practice for family therapists was to work in live supervision teams. Specifically, they addressed the dilemmas of family therapists and systemic practitioners who wanted the perceived advantages of incorporating a meta-perspective into their work, but who did not have access to technology such as video suites and one-way screens, who may have worked in people's homes, or in residential accommodation, or who worked primarily on their own. They suggested working in pairs, not as co-therapists, but as a lead therapist and an in-room consultant. The in-room consultant can both take the notes of the meeting and offer live consultation, i.e. making comments directly to the therapist, which are heard by the family members, who then have the chance to comment further. This strategy leaves the therapist in the more central position in relation to the family members and able to incorporate the consultant's suggestions into the flow of therapy. In addition, the therapist is able to lean into the consultant and ask for his or her views and suggestions, both to enhance the development of ideas and to effect progress when the therapist is feeling stuck with the therapeutic process.

In Kingston and Smith's approach, in-room consultation afforded particular opportunities to support the therapy and the family's members in their efforts to develop understanding and make changes in their lives, and to provide live training supervision for a less experienced therapist. For example, the consultant could support the therapy by suggesting a specific focus, or by seeking further information, offering reframing and suggesting alternative solutions to those being considered by the therapist and family members; could support the therapist in training by helping him or her to return to a focus which has been lost, identifying issues not recognized by the therapist, and balancing the therapist's bias if an unhelpful coalition with some family members seems to be developing; and could support the family by endorsing what is going well and offering understanding for their dilemmas.

Kingston and Smith used a break near the end of the therapy meeting in which the therapist and the in-room consultant would take their leave of the family, briefly, to discuss the work and perhaps to develop a summary message to offer the family members. Given that it has been questioned whether it is necessary to exclude the family members from this process of therapeutic summarizing, we shall refer to the work of Vetere and Cooper (2001), who further developed the approach of in-room consultation in the Reading Safer Families Project when working systemically with family violence.

Similarly to Kingston and Smith, Vetere and Cooper use the in-room consultant role to support what is going well, to acknowledge success where it may have been overlooked, to reflect on the therapeutic process, to comment on a difficulty or sadness without offering a solution, to introduce new ideas, and to ask confrontational or challenging questions in ways that facilitate constructive problem-solving. This ability to work in partnership is crucial when addressing accountability for violent behaviour, challenging the perpetrator/s and creating a context for safety in family relationships.

Vetere and Cooper develop their ideas in conversation with each other in front of the family, as part of the therapeutic process. The therapist invites reflections from the in-room consultant on what has transpired between the family and the therapist, and invites family members to comment on what has been said. Thus, all participants are invited to adopt the roles of speaker, listener, and observer, and to comment on differences and similarities in perceptions. Vetere and Cooper have few rules for the in-room consultant, which include always being brief, not using too many ideas, being tentative, and always encouraging family members to comment on their ideas. Thus, the therapy pair is accountable publicly for their thinking and the development of their ideas in practice. Vetere and Cooper use their method of reflecting practice in a more informal way when attending network meetings and reviews, when acting as consultants to professional workers, teams, and organizations, and when writing their reports. David Amias (2001, personal communication) and his colleagues, working in a Child and Adolescent Mental Health Services (CAMHS) team, use reflection when discussing team policy and strategy at their regular meetings. On a rotating basis, two team members sit "outside" the team discussion, and then reflect for ten minutes, near the end of the meeting, while their colleagues listen. David Amias reports that it has helped team members to avoid symmetrical escalations around conflictual issues and to remain thoughtful around issues that arouse passionate feelings, and seems to guarantee a voice for points of view that might ordinarily struggle to be heard in the face of strong opinions and vested interests.

We do not want to suggest that reflecting practices are straightforward. There are pitfalls for the unwary in these approaches, as in any others. Vetere and Cooper (2001) point out that therapist/consultant pairs have to work hard to develop a smooth working process. Aiming at more open and straightforward discussion in therapeutic work also affects their relationship, in terms of what they do and do not say to each other. Success is seen as a question of fit, timing, and process, with a constant eye on the tension between the constraints and benefits of this type of working. Both sides of the pair share a mutual responsibility to challenge the other to avoid a fall into a "*folie a deux*", while staying alert to the darker forces of envy, rivalry, and competition (for example, to say the most clever thing, or have the family members remember and value more the contribution from one side of the pair), which would ensure that the purpose is no longer helpful to the family. The in-room consultant needs to learn fast when to avoid an intervention; for example, when it interrupts the development of a theme, or risks overwhelming the family.

In the context of live supervision of family therapy using a one-way screen and an observing team, the work of Andersen (1987) has been most influential in promoting more transparent practices. Instead of consulting in relative isolation to an anonymous and potentially oppressive supervision team, the discussions between the therapist and team are held openly in front of the family. One variant in practice is for the supervising team to discuss their reflections of the therapy while the therapist and family members "listen in". Arguably, the supervision team is not imposing interventions, including new meanings and beliefs, on families, but are sharing their thoughts and concerns with them. This is not to pretend that a thought "offered" by a team member may not be "heard" as advice or an "instruction", given the nature of a help-seeking relationship with those who have expertise. However, through the team's discussions, the family members are invited to consider alternative explanations, stories, and attributions regarding their lives together. At times, the reflecting team may disagree and debate different possible ideas and explanations among themselves. This may allow different family members who hold opposing views to feel understood, and may perhaps enable them to move on to more constructive points of view. Importantly, the reflecting team enables family members to hear, and perhaps begin to internalize, a different conversation rather than simply different explanations. By being able to internalize different conversations they are, in Bateson's (1980) terms, "learning to learn", or being encouraged to become more creative. The therapy thereby becomes less concerned with content and less in danger of being marooned in attempts to offer families a "better" view or story.

Another variant to more transparent live consultation can be found in Andy Treacher's (personal communication) early attempts to use a speakerphone to transmit messages from the supervising team, so that all could hear what was being said to the therapist, or to send in, with permission, a team member to the therapy room to discuss the team's developing ideas with the therapist and family. Some therapists (White, 1995) also engage in more or less open discussion of political issues, such as the oppressive nature of discourses of mental health, and assist family members to resist through "externalizing" their problems. Instead of viewing problems as being due to personal failing, people are encouraged to resist, with the therapist's assistance, the dilemmas and contradictions contained, for example, in some dominant notions of mental health such as, unemotionality, self-sufficiency, non-vulnerability, independence, stability, and so on. Manojlovic and Partridge (2001) offer a clear description of how they use systemic ideas to challenge some of these notions when working in acute adult psychiatric settings.

As we can see, the use of the reflecting team and reflective processes offers a variety of narratives that invite family members perhaps to think in different ways and to choose what might make a better fit for them. Apart from the content of the discussion, they may experience a different process of conversation, for example in hearing the reflecting team discussing potentially difficult and conflictual issues in a less emotional way. In a sense this can be viewed as a form of modelling, but the process is less directive and more collaborative in its intent.

Reflexive notes

1. Can you identify any gendered beliefs from your childhood? What are your ideas about how men and women *should* be changing? How do these beliefs and ideas affect your practice now? Note in this exercise the pervasive power of the word *should* in holding a normalizing gaze or mirror in which we are reminded of our defects and *abnormality*.
2. In discussion with a trusted colleague, or in a peer supervision group, you might like to explore the following questions and ideas:

   (a) think, for example, about your name—where does it come from? what are the cultural connections? what stories are told in your family about your name and its connections, such as, about temperament and culture, religion, life styles;
   (b) brainstorm and unpack the meanings held in the phrase "Universality that exists in diversity", and consider how these meanings impact on your practice as a clinician;
   (c) what has changed in your culture over the last twenty years? What are the cultural norms that we find difficult—how do we decide where we draw the line? How do you talk to clients about the potential benefits or harms within certain cultural practices?
   (d) what are your motivations for working with families living in minority groups? How does your own ethnic background inform how you work with families across different ethnic groupings?

CHAPTER SIX

Specific applications: integrative practice—context and method

This section explores some of the applications of systemic ideas and practices across a range of service settings and with specific issues.

Working systemically with couples

The work of Zimmerman and Dickerson (1993) will be described in some detail as it illustrates nicely an attempt to converge social constructionism, family systems thinking, and second order cybernetics with White and Epston's (1990) ideas as a narrative model for working with couples. This posits that people choose specific incidents from their past experience to justify and explain their present behaviour, constructing meanings which become small stories, scripts, and myths (Bruner, 1990). It is suggested that any new events that confirm or conform to the story are added over time, so that the stories become treated as if true, and people can be influenced by them or act in accordance with them. Some accounts we hold are said to be problem-saturated. At first sight, this model seems to suggest that people are not reflective, or that they do not notice disconfirming events. Rather, the model suggests that people's accounts and explanations can be influenced by prevailing socialization processes, gender training, cultural, economic, and political conditions, that may operate outside full conscious attention. Zimmerman and Dickerson's model suggests that couples' reciprocal patterns of interaction connect both the socially constructed meanings and the habits of the couple. It does not assume, however, that partners in a couple relationship have equity in their relationship and equal influence on these patterns.

In therapy, the couple are invited to describe reciprocal patterns of interaction that constrain their relationship and to explore the different discourses that might be said to support these patterns. As in most psychotherapies, the purpose is to help the partners distance themselves from these patterns, psychologically speaking, and to try to develop other descriptions of themselves and their relationship that also are grounded in their experience. So, in narrative terms, the therapy becomes a process within which existing patterns and prevailing discourses are deconstructed while simultaneous restorying is taking place along preferred lines.

The process of therapy moves through joining with the couple and establishing the therapeutic relationship, externalizing the problem or problems, using relative influence questioning, exploring discourses that support the problem or problems, and responding to the new story. The process of joining described here has much in common with the practice of structural therapists (Minuchin, 1974) and Haley's (1976) writing about the first interview with a family. The emphasis is very much on social aspects, i.e., getting to know people as people, rather than clients, first, putting them at their ease, finding out about their interests and competencies, before beginning a more detailed exploration of their problems and concerns.

When the conversation moves into problem talk, each partner is asked to describe how they experience the problem, with an emphasis on understanding the reciprocal nature of their interaction. This approach draws heavily on early family systems' thinking, which seeks to understand the nature of relational patterns and how they are maintained over time. A common cycle described by couples would be one of "approach/avoidance" or "nag/withdraw", i.e., one partner perceives a wrong or a problem and seeks a solution, the other partner experiences the approach as criticizing and defensively withdraws. The withdrawal may be perceived as stonewalling, and the approaching partner redoubles his or her efforts in an attempt to elicit the desired response. Such a cycle of interaction can escalate into a row, or a period of silence, within which little movement or creative thinking seems to take place. It is not difficult to see, in this example, how the couple are "prevented" from solving their problems. Exploration and externalization of such interactional cycles would pay careful attention to gender-related themes and other contextual factors that impinge on the couple's relationship. When describing these sequences, Zimmerman and Dickerson (1993) prefer the phrase "reciprocal invitation" to "circular causal behaviour" because it seems to keep open the possibility of other choices; for example, turning down the invitation to participate in the usual way.

A few caveats are in order. When working with high conflict and abusive behaviour, it is important to establish safety first, and clear grounds for accountability for the perpetrators of harm and the therapeutic practice, before embarking on a systemic analysis that might appear to hold a victim equally responsible for abusive cycles of behaviour. Later in this chapter we offer a more complete description of this approach to working with violent behaviour.

Some couples are less able to give clear descriptions of their interactive sequences, and rather than struggle to establish them, it might be more helpful to the couple to externalize aspects of their life-style that they find unhelpful, such as, what the reciprocal habits are on which this lifestyle is based. It is likely that this will lead to a discussion of beliefs or expectations that might be said to underpin their behavioural choices and, at this point, careful tracking of these beliefs will facilitate later exploration of behavioural sequences.

Some couples might wish to present a symptom such as anxiety, for discussion. Using this approach you can track the effects of anxiety on their relationship together, on each other, and so on, in a way that can lead to the construction of patterns. Similarly, if a partner or couple is highly distressed, you can track the effects of such distress, and then notice the difference with other aspects of their relationship where they report different experiences. In this way, you can more easily focus on the patterns that support the distress without seeming persecutory to the couple.

Questioning processes, or relative influence questioning, as

Zimmerman and Dickerson (1993) prefer to say, is the therapist's means of using curiosity to explore carefully how the defined problem has influence over people's choices, relationships, and so on. Both partners fully participate in this questioning process, while the therapist broadens the questions to explore points of entry to other solutions, such as times when the problem has less effect, or contexts in which the problem is not present. For example, shyness in a relationship might be experienced differently in different settings, with others present or absent, or in other relationships. These questions are designed to help people notice and pay more attention to the times when the problem is less of a problem, i.e., when they escape the pattern.

Let us consider Jim and May, who started to talk to their therapist about their wish to be more emotionally intimate with each other. They seemed to agree that there was an emotional distance between them, despite their strong commitment to each other and their marriage. They explored, with the help of their therapist, what might have been some formative earlier experiences that underpinned their ideas about themselves and their relationship. May said that she had experienced emotional intimacy in friendships with other women, and thus had a good sense of what she was seeking with Jim. Jim, however, found it hard to identify experiences of emotional intimacy in his other relationships. As they talked further, they identified some current patterns in their interaction that seemed to characterize their sense of emotional distance, such as, if Jim perceived May as critical when she asked him to respond to her at an emotional level, he would withdraw. They escaped this pattern at least once in their meeting with their therapist, who was able to pause and notice this different sequence and then invite them to reflect on their experience of it. Thus, while Jim was talking about his sense of emotional distance from others, he began to weep. May moved towards him and comforted him with a hug, telling him she loved him. He turned into the hug and stayed with it for a few moments. When May moved back to her chair, their therapist asked them to reflect on their experience. What they both noticed was that prior to these discussions, at a point of vulnerability Jim would not have allowed himself to accept May's comfort. He would have perceived it to be a criticism of his ability to cope, and a threat to his own view of himself (Figure 1).

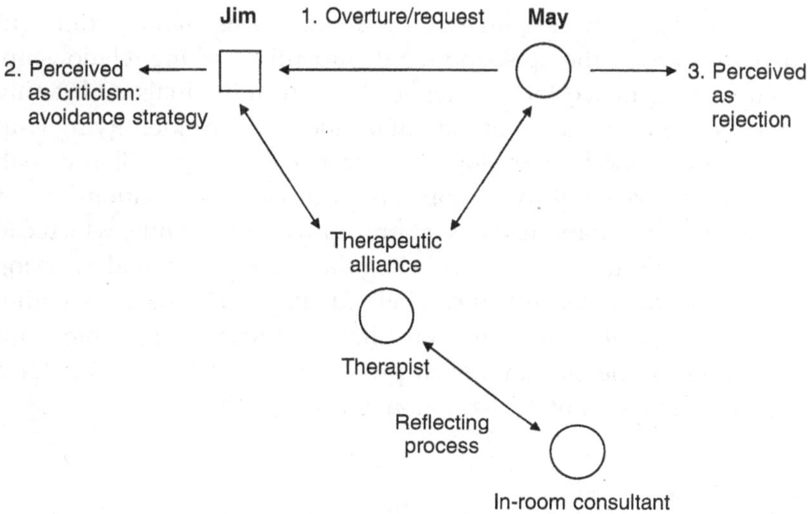

Figure 1. Escaping a fixed pattern of behaviour with the help of a therapeutic alliance.

Zimmerman and Dickerson (1993) describe the process of responding to the new story as a gentle and persistent way of helping the couple take small steps away from the problem, while continuing to look for competence and examples of escaping the pattern. They recommend talking to each partner directly about the steps they have made. At the same time, the therapist is exploring the beliefs that constrain choice, such as in our example above, the fear or dislike of criticism as a motive for avoiding straight talking. Their approach holds some curiosity about the origins of these beliefs, for example, in previous relationship experiences, or in family-of-origin relationships. Such exploration is facilitated by a strong, empathic, therapeutic relationship, and helps the therapist move quickly, when necessary, to discussion of experiences that highlight alternative, more constructive beliefs as a challenge to constraining beliefs and discourses. In conclusion, Zimmerman and Dickerson argue that therapy which begins with looking at behavioural patterns often ends up with a careful consideration of aspects of relationship discourse that have been around for a long time in people's lives, as we saw in the example with Jim and May.

Working with couples can be described as making different demands on the therapist and the therapeutic working relationship, compared with working systemically with individuals and family groups. For example, common pitfalls include over-identifying with one partner and/or developing a stronger working alliance with one partner, leading to an unbalanced therapeutic relationship, or experiencing a triangulated relationship with the couple, which can create unhelpful dependencies. Regular supervision and working with an in-room consultant can help identify such processes within the therapy, and in-room consultation provides a vehicle for reflecting on the effects of such processes. (See Chapter One for a further discussion of triangulation and couple dyads.)

Working systemically with individuals

It is not surprising that less has been written overall about the usefulness of systemic ideas and practices when working with individuals because, after all, the systemic tradition grew out of thinking about relationships and how individual distress could be seen at one level of explanation not as an attribute of an individual, but rather as an emergent property of relationships. Thus, the field grew out of an energetic pursuit of ideas and methods that helped individuals in relation to one another, at work, at home, in institutions, in friendship, in sickness, and so on. However, on reflection, it might be seen as odd to have neglected this dimension of systemic practice, as many family therapists and systemic practitioners see individuals as adjunctive practice in the context of family work, or as individual work in its own right. But they do not seem to write about it. There are some notable exceptions, such as Jenkins and Asen (1992) and Boscolo and Bertrando (1996), writing for a general systemic audience, or Jones (1991) and Jenkins (1990), writing for practitioners who work respectively with survivors of sexual abuse and with men who behave violently. We suspect that the earlier, historical attempts to define the boundaries of systemic working as different to prevailing work in behavioural methods and psychodynamic methods, long before the cognitive revolution in psychology, contributed to a reluctance to be seen on paper to commit to working with individuals.

It may be a reflection of maturity in the field that the wider applications of systemic thinking and the clear rapprochement with other psychotherapeutic methods and approaches facilitates a growing literature on working systemically with individuals. In an earlier section, we have explored some of the benefits of these recent (and not so recent) attempts at integrative practice. We would argue that many mental health practitioners have rarely been purist in their approach, always preferring to formulate their thinking within explanatory frameworks that best fit the difficulties at hand. Thus, an approach to working with individuals that facilitates loyalty to preferred models and methods and, at the same time, provides an overarching conceptual framework that enables reflexive thinking about the connections between ideas and between ideas and practices, would appeal to many mental health practitioners. Systemic practice with individuals can fit into such a frame. We shall outline some ideas and practices that we have found helpful when working systemically with individuals.

Arguably, the most important aspect of this work is to think systemically and to maintain a reflexive stance in relation to the work. The focus of the work will be more on the social and political context of the person, the relationships they inhabit, the iterative effects of living in relationship to others, whatever the context, and the connections between the person and events, beliefs and behaviours, of the context under study. This puts the person's problems in a larger framework, with multiple levels of explanation possible and more choice as to which level of intervention to select. The range of options for ensuring a good fit between the explanations and the interventions has been expanded.

Although other people may not participate in the therapy, they are always in the thinking of both the therapist and the client and are thus alive in the therapy room. The effect of the therapist on the client's other relationships, and the effects of others on the therapist–client relationship are always attended to and discussed, actively mirroring the notion that any two people's relationship is always responsive to a third, who may not be present. Any changes promoted in therapy, or achieved, are always reviewed for their effects on the client's other relationships, as well as on their relationship with themselves, so to speak. Thus, the client is helped to remain oriented towards relationships and resources in the world, rather than using the intensity of the transference relationship *per se* as the vehicle for change, whereas the therapist tries to maintain a reflexive position within the therapeutic discourse and to elicit and discuss the client's beliefs about therapy.

Systemic theories of change are as helpful when working with individuals as when working with couples and family groups. Key points to consider are as follows.

- Understanding beliefs about personal "stuckness" in terms of repeated attempted solutions to a problem, which become the problem in their own right. So, is "symptomatic" behaviour a result of a solution that has backfired? (Watzlawick *et al.*, 1974) For example, in a *Peanuts* cartoon, we see Snoopy sitting on the hockey bench, waiting for his turn to play in the match. He's feeling anxious and decides to tape his hockey stick as a solution to his anxiety—a calming activity. However, Snoopy manages to tape himself to the stick and the stick to the bench, ending up in a completely messy ball of black sticky tape. Thus, the attempted solution to the problem of Snoopy's anxiety becomes the problem of becoming taped to the hockey bench.
- We might query whether the "symptomatic" behaviour is an ironic consequence of previous attempts to adapt and stabilize around changes in relationships? A typical example in work with an individual who is experiencing distress regarding their relationship may be when she has attempted to solve this by spending more time on her own. However, the effects of this attempted solution can be that she then starts to feel increasingly isolated and desperately worried that her relationship is deteriorating.
- Does the behaviour seem to serve some function for the family as a whole; for example, how would family members be stressed if the person were to change? (Selvini-Palazzoli *et al.*, 1980b). Is it possible that the individual with the "symptomatic" behaviour might be acting out someone else's upset? (Scharff & Scharff, 1987).
- Does the symptomatic behaviour seem to prevent an expected or unwanted life-cycle change, however ironically, and who might seem to benefit most from these changes not happening as expected? (Carter & McGoldrick, 1989).

Chris

> Chris, a young man aged 16, living with his twin brother and single-parent mother, was increasingly developing a drug abuse problem. This could be seen both as an attempt to gain some independence from his mother and as maintaining his dependence and inability to separate. At times he was so "out of it" on drugs (mainly cannabis) and sometimes alcohol that he could be sure that his mother's anxieties would be activated about whether he might come to harm, for example when he went out on the town. In contrast to many other adolescents, Chris made no attempt to disguise his drug usage from his mother. In a sense his behaviour almost appeared to be inviting his mother's anxious and concerned responses. His behaviour and his mother's reactions could be seen within the wider context of his mother's feelings of guilt about having left Chris with his father when he was aged 8. In effect, it seemed that Chris's behaviour in part kept him dependent on his mother and in a way provided the opportunity for her to "prove" to herself that she was a "good " and caring mother. In individual therapy Chris revealed that he did quite like the care and attention his mother showed him and that he was aware that his actions would invite her concern, despite his initial protests that all he wanted was for her to stop "fussing and going on at him".

Systemic theories of change do not assume that the initiating conditions for the development of the problematic behaviour are the same as the maintaining conditions, which is very similar to the operating assumptions of a functional analysis. The difference is subtle, and lies in the direction of causality, in that a functional analysis might take a more linear approach, and systemic is more circular and iterative, with the primary emphases on the feedback loop and the reflexive position of the observer, rather than the behavioural consequences *per se*.

Systemic work with individuals is usually short-term. Sessions might be widely spaced, and tasks and rituals might be negotiated, both individual and systems oriented, for work inside and outside the therapeutic sessions. For example, working with a woman and a mother who experienced a profound depression, it seemed the depression experience was linked to an unacknowledged and private grief. The woman had given birth to a stillborn child, following a difficult pregnancy, in which she felt very ambiguous about on the one hand wanting the unborn child and; on the other, at times actively wishing she was not pregnant. The birth of her dead child had confirmed that she was being punished for thinking "poisonous" thoughts about her child, and that in some way she had killed her baby. In the therapy, the mother had been encouraged to find a polaroid photograph of her child, taken by the hospital. She and her husband subsequently decided to have a local artist paint a portrait of the child from the photograph, which was to be placed on their living room wall. This action was key in signalling to other family members and relatives that it was possible to talk about the baby. It would seem that they had remained silent for fear of upsetting the mother further and exacerbating her depression. Following the family unveiling of the portrait, the mother and her husband decided to hold a memorial service for their dead child, to which they invited their relatives and friends. These rituals of remembrance and celebration broke the silence around the dead child, and seemed to signal the lifting of the mother's depression and her improved ability to take up the threads of her life again.

The past may well be explored, not in its own right, but more as the context within which to explore and reframe current patterns, develop new meanings, and create new narratives. The use of circular questioning and reframing can be helpful, as can more active interventions, such as role play, role reversal, and sculpting as visual ways of portraying patterns and identifying constraints and possible solutions. Genograms are useful devices for exploring an individual's idiosyncratic world view, particularly of the intergenerational transmission of family-wide beliefs, patterns, and practices (McGoldrick & Gersen, 1989). In many ways a genogram can act like a projective test, garnering information about a person's implicit and explicit assumptions, wishes, fears, and values.

Meeting the cast of characters not in therapy, with your client's consent, is another active way of helping to reconstruct the past and help choose therapeutic directions; for example, towards changing or accepting relationships. A one-off consultation with one or more significant others, such as partners, adult siblings, and so on, can be very helpful to individual therapists. Such meetings can help correct a tendency to blame, help make the system more hospitable to individual change, and help the therapist understand their client's interactional style from another perspective. Preparation for such a meeting can often include a thoughtful look at the genogram, with the questioning organized around others' relationship to both the individual and the problematic issues.

Predicting a relapse as an approach to prevention and the maintenance of change has much in common with motivational interviewing, but goes one step further in considering the systemic consequences of both relapse and change. Systemically oriented therapists are interested in resilience and seek out strengths and resources, possibly underutilized, including the subjugated accounts of self, and the logical meanings for problematic behaviour. This is usually a matter of emphasis, in that negative or adverse feelings are acknowledged and explored, but not highlighted as much as they might be in other approaches. Wider system constraints and resources, such as relative wealth, gender, class-based issues, religious beliefs, and wider cultural constraints and affordances are explored, often with the help of a genogram to orchestrate some of the demographic information and its social, relational and psychological impacts.

Systemically-minded therapists are usually prepared to work towards clients' goals within a collaborative frame, unless, for example, there is a moral issue at stake about the use of violence and other methods of abuse to have an effect in the world and get one's own way. We shall say more about working with violent behaviour later in this section.

Systemic consultation to families and professionals

Brunning and Huffington (1990) defined consultancy as a direct or indirect process enabling individuals, groups, or organizations to fulfil their role, functions, or tasks better. It is a process by which the persons seeking consultation ask for help in identifying and clarifying concerns and in considering the options available for problem resolution. Thus, the consultees retain the legal, ethical, and administrative responsibility for initiative and action, unlike supervision, where there may well be a hierarchical relationship between the supervisor and supervisee, or therapy, where there may be pressure to accept suggestions in pursuit of therapeutic effectiveness.

Street, Downey, and Brazier

Consultation for families may well be a prologue to therapy, or a feasible alternative to therapy. Street *et al.*, (1991) describe an approach to family consultation that both screens for the appropriateness of therapy and offers a forum to discuss concerns and seek advice and reassurance. They adapted the 2+1 model of therapy developed by Barkham (1989), whereby they would offer a family two meetings about two weeks apart, and then a follow-up meeting three months later. The follow-up meeting was intended to provide a safety net if the issues had not been resolved within the context of the first two meetings. They audited their service and found that only one out of every five families referred to their child psychology service necessitated a longer-term course of family therapy.

Their approach within the first two meetings drew on some systemic and Winnicottian ideas of consultation, the "interpretative method" (Bateson, 1980), and the use of the written word in the form of letter writing (White & Epston, 1990). Winnicott (1971) often saw children once, partly in response to circumstances of high social need and scarce resources. He was concerned to "loosen the knot of the developmental process" and facilitate some improvement in symptomatic behaviour. According to Winnicott, the task of the consultant is to communicate understanding to the child in such a way that there is a merging between the child's positive expectations of the helper and the actual helper. Such confirmation of the child allows the consultant to enhance the child's confidence in some developmental movement.

Street *et al.* also draw on Bateson's ideas that interactions and behaviours are determined by the different meanings that family members attribute to events and relationships. Based on the systemic idea that family groups evolve their own unique patterns of behaviour over time, it is thought these patterns can be described either as a result of behavioural observation, or by asking questions that tap into the family members' consensual view of their immediate circumstances. The questions are asked in a way that promotes new possibilities. Street *et al.* quote Andersen (1987) who suggests that this process occurs at three levels: (1) the account family members offer of their world, enlarged by the process of the therapist building an understanding of the family's understanding; (2) the process of family members and the therapist together developing an explanatory account for how the family's circumstances arose; and (3) the ways in which the therapist tries to help create a context wherein family members can entertain alternative explanations and predictions for the future.

In addition, Street *et al.* draw on elements of the literary tradition by writing letters to the family as support for therapeutic change. They communicate their ideas about the family's problem both orally during the first two meetings, and as a written communication after those meetings. They try to write a straightforward letter in which they outline their opinions and possible future actions.

Their model of consultation is a synthesis of the above three traditions, delivered within the 2+1 model described above. During their therapeutic consultations they try to establish: (a) an interactive view of the referral process; (b) an interactive view of the problem; (c) the family's ideology of the problem; and (d) the family members' expectations of the consultant and the process of consultation. Their audit of the consultation meetings within a community child psychology service suggested that people came to them with five sets of expectations, broadly speaking: (1) we are here because professional X wanted us to come; (2) we wanted your views on him/her/us; (3) we were hoping for some advice or guidelines for the problem; (4) we thought you would talk to our child and find out the reasons why he/she is behaving this way; and (5) we hoped that by talking to you we would find the best way of dealing with this problem. Street *et al.* concluded from their audit that the latter expectation represented an invitation for therapy, whereas the first four expectations were an invitation to consultation.

Wynne, McDaniel, and Weber

Similarly, Wynne *et al.*, (1986) describe consultation with families as a process whereby they assume family members' abilities for responsible decision-making, and family resources and competence are directly tapped. Decisions about whom to invite to the consultation meetings are largely organized by participants' perceptions of where the impasse in the system occurs. Importantly, the systemic view of consultation would locate the consultant as a necessary part of the system requiring consultation.

Wynne *et al.*, (1986) propose a model of systems consultation, informed by structural and strategic ideas, which they argue is applicable to working with teams and organizations. They have described the stages in their approach to consultation as *exploring, contracting, connecting, assessing, implementing, evaluating,* and *leaving*. The stages are not mutually exclusive and are intended only as a process guide for the consultant.

Exploring involves both clarifying the request for consultation and identifying exactly who is requesting the consultation, by considering how the request came about, why you were asked, who approves the request, and the role and position of the consultee in the team or organization requesting the consultation. In particular, it is helpful to consider the potential political ramifications of the request for consultation, including any personal or professional investment you may have in the success or failure of the consultation.

Contracting is the process whereby agreement is reached on the goals of the consultation, the services provided by the consultant, the procedures for sharing information, and other practical arrangements, such as the venue. Consideration of the risks and consequences of the consultation is also part of the process. At this stage it is important to be clear about whom else might be working with the consultee or team, such as supervisors, administrators, managers, and even other consultants, whose influence will have an effect on the process of consultation.

Connecting is the process of engaging key members of the consultation system in the consultation process and deciding how and when they will be involved in goal-setting.

Assessing refers to the methods by which you gather information and the systemic and other theoretical concepts used to understand the organization's structure, function, and dynamics. The assessment process focuses on organizational life-cycle issues, the important relational dynamics within the system, such as hierarchies, coalitions, triangles, and boundary problems, recent events triggering the consultation request, previous attempted solutions to the problem, and the belief systems of the consultees.

Implementing involves specifying the systemic interventions chosen to meet the consultation request, making decisions about whether education is provided, deciding the means of collaborating with the consultees over implementation, and choosing the procedures to ensure the maintenance of change. It is important that the implementation methods are consistent with the organization's belief systems, and that any new goals which emerged during the consultation process have also been addressed.

Evaluating is the process of deciding how the consultation goals and organizational changes have been met, who will take part in the evaluation process, planning for follow-up evaluation, and allowing time and opportunity to reflect on the consultation process itself.

Leaving describes the means by which a consultation is ended, or the consultant negotiates a new contract for a new problem or a different role within the organization.

Losing our way as a consultant is one of the most common pitfalls. Wynne *et al.* identify some of these pitfalls and offer advice to the unwary. Taking time to clarify in particular the nature of the contract, the consultant role, and the goals and desired outcomes of the consultation, can go a long way towards avoiding contractual misunderstandings. This advice is often offered as "look before you leap", similar to the advice offered to those who work with complex organizational networks and convene and chair network meetings. Hidden agendas are thought by many to be part of the process of any request for consultation, so the consultant needs to move lightly within the explicit agenda and keep alert to the possibility of covert processes and goals. Mapping the system under consultation, looking at patterns of relationship, communication, and feedback, within and across hierarchies, can often identify points where more implicit concerns might emerge. This mapping process can help clarify the extent to which people are going through the motions and are not really committed to the process of consultation. If this proved to be the case, it would impede meaningful goal-planning and implementation.

Occasionally a consultee or team of people requesting a consultation may be receiving help from a number of sources, known and unknown. It is always helpful to track sources of support, advice, and reassurance within and outside the system to try to avoid a complex clash of interests and direction when goal-planning. One of the responsibilities of the consultant, similar to that of a therapist, is to prepare the system under consultation for some of the probable systemic consequences of the consultation, such as changes to the organization of the system, people's roles, and modes and means of communication. Finally, we should note the tendency for a consultant and an organization to become comfortable with the consultant's presence, perhaps resulting in the work being unnecessarily prolonged. It is helpful to plan the end of the consultation from the beginning, asking ourselves questions such as, "What needs to happen for me/them to know this piece of work is finished?". This does not preclude further consultation or follow-up visits, but warns of the dangers of becoming another member of staff, so to speak!

David Campbell

In contrast to the model described above, Campbell (1995) offers an alternative model of systemic consultation, specifically designed to help other family therapists who are "stuck" in their clinical work with a family. He adapts the Milan systemic model of family therapy to this task, using theoretical concepts of meaning, pattern, recursiveness, and difference. He treats requests for consultation much like a referral about a family and hypothesizes about the way the problem has led to the group feeling stuck, and the wider meaning that "being stuck" might have for the family and team in their community and neighbourhood groupings. He is alert to the problem of the request for consultation being part of the failed attempt to find a solution, and so tries to create a space within which people can feel safe enough to make new connections and broaden the context in which they made the initial request.

The consultation interview follows a similar procedure to a Milan-style family interview, with pre-session hypothesizing based on preliminary information, the use of circular questioning and reframing, characterized by the neutral stance of the therapist, and with mid-session breaks for discussion and final formulation. The main aim of this style of consultation is to provide a space to comment on and clarify some of the confusions that arise when working in systems where different meanings for behaviour arise from the differing perspectives from which that behaviour is viewed. In an interesting variation, Campbell writes of the advantages of asking consultees to play each other's roles, following scripted versions based on earlier information gathering. This allows a discussion where people get close to the issues that concern them, listen to others' points of view, and all within the safety of being in a role. They can play with new ideas and new ways of approaching their difficulties within a situation that closely resembles their own.

Campbell and his colleagues have developed their consultation model to include the management of change within organizations, and the facilitation of interdisciplinary working relationships (Campbell, 1995; Campbell, 2001; Campbell *et al.*, 1991). They are interested in exploring how individuals might work more effectively within organizations. They use ideas from the fields of constructivism and social constructionism alongside their core concept of the organizational life-cycle to address the interpretation of meaning at all levels of the system's structure. In particular, they reflect on the potential conflict between ideas held at individual, group, and organizational levels and the process of developing connections between these differing meaning systems. One aim is to facilitate changes in the meaning systems within the wider organization. Campbell and his colleagues outline a seven-stage model for consultation within organizations that helps teams and wider systems to learn to become observers of their own process and their own organization as a means to initiating such changes.

In summary, then, some of the problems associated with systems consultation include: (a) understanding the limitations and risks for consultation in terms of wider societal needs; (b) limitations on purchasing and providing consultation within a modern managed health-care system; (c) the lack of relevant research showing the potential for consultancy to broach wider questions of economic and political circumstances as they impact on peoples' lives; and (d) potential difficulties in defining the boundaries of the system under consultation. Conversely, some of the advantages include: (a) the consultation process does not prejudge the nature of the problem and facilitates the development of collaborative relationships; (b) consultation facilitates the use of reframing, and provides a context for identifying and exploring sources of resilience and other interpersonal resources; (c) the consultant is both part of the system under consultation and in a meta-position, and thus is able to assess relationships and patterns; and (d) the consultant role does not preclude a shift to an alternative professional role; for example, when consultation to a family is a precursor to therapy.

Working with violence in family relationships

> People are more likely to be killed, physically assaulted, hit, beaten up, slapped or spanked in their own homes by other family members than anywhere else, or by anyone else in our society. [Gelles & Cornell, 1990]

Working with couples and families where physical violence is known or suspected to be happening is a serious and worrying affair. We believe that people have the right to live without intimidation, threat or fear of harm, and actual harm. If we are to prioritize safety in family members' relationships and hold responsible those who harm others, we need to be clear about our own moral position on the use of violence and our relationship to the means of social control if the violent behaviour does not cease. Physical assault is a criminal offence.

Minimization and denial of violent behaviour and the effects of violence on intimate relationships is endemic (Hearn, 1994). If we are to guard against inadvertent support for the cultural beliefs and practices that maintain violent patterns of behaviour and do not challenge their occurrence, we need to examine our own beliefs, theories, and prejudices about the use of violence in intimate relationships and develop clear individual and organizational policies to help us in developing our own approaches to safe practice. This is no mean task. We write this section to encourage and support you as you engage with this serious topic, which is, after all, a topic that touches all of us. In writing this section, we draw heavily on the work of Vetere and Cooper (2001, 2003) in the Reading Safer Families project.

The nature and complexity of the problem

The British Crime Survey (1996) identified 30% of all reported violent crime to be domestic assault, with 90% of women reporting attacks by their male partners, and 48% of men reporting attacks by their female partners. The attacks by men are reported to be more frequent and more severe. The same survey published in 2000 identified 23% of assaults as occurring between people living in domestic relationships. The rate of repeat victimization was highest for domestic violence, with 57% of the sample of 23% reporting at least two incidents within the survey year. Writing in the USA, Straus and Gelles (1990) estimated that one in eight women were seriously physically assaulted by their male partner each year, and that one in three women were seriously assaulted over the course of their relationship. Under-reporting is widely believed to be a problem, with estimates ranging from one-third to two out of ninety-eight assaults under-reported (Dobash & Dobash, 1992).

Moffitt and Caspi (1998), in their review of the effects on children of witnessing adult violence, estimate that adult partners who are violent to each other are four to nine times more likely to be violent to their children. The NSPCC (1985) estimated that ninety-nine children died of non-accidental injury in the year of their survey, but that they had underestimated by one half. Browne and Herbert (1997) reported that in 1997 the cost of direct medical services to the victims of family violence in the USA was $44 million. This figure did not include the immediate costs of policing or social services. The wider costs of undetected violence include the long-term effects of pushing, shoving, and slapping on self-esteem and psychological well-being, the potential for so-called minor violence to escalate, and the effects on the children caught up in the violence. Known violence from one family member to another is often an indicator of a relational context of intimidation, coercion, and fear, which can make therapeutic change difficult if the perpetrator of violence does not take responsibility for their behaviour.

It would appear that couples and family counsellors and therapists may not ask routinely about acts of violence in intimate relationships, nor, it seems, do therapists and counsellors who work with adolescents ask about dating violence, nor do they ask children about whether there is violence at home. Not only would such information help in formulating around troubled and troubling behaviour, but not asking makes it more likely that clients will not tell (Ehrensaft & Vivian, 1996; Straus, 1994). Ehrensaft and Vivian, in their sample of 136 couples, found that 60% had experienced violent assault in the year preceding counselling, but only 10% spontaneously reported the violence to their counsellor. When asked why they did not tell, the clients' list of reasons was long: perceiving physical violence to be trivial and tolerable; not the "real" problem; fearing further victimization; feelings of shame; wanting to make a good impression; love and concern for the partner; and so on. The counsellors' reasons were that they did not ask and that it was not part of their assessment procedure! We would suggest that we do need to find a way to ask routinely about behaviours that harm and otherwise threaten safety, both psychological and physical.

The effects on children of witnessing violence

Moffitt and Caspi (1998) estimate that at least two-thirds of household assaults are witnessed by children. Some children are known to be at risk of traumatic responses and heightened risk of internalizing and externalizing problems. The frequency and intensity of the physical conflict between the parents is often linked to worse behavioural outcomes for children. Browne and Herbert (1997) speculate that mediating mechanisms might include disruption to parenting, stress for children and the disruption of their security, the tendency for children to imitate their parent's behaviour, learning that violence is normative and that people get away with it. In addition, repeated exposure of children to violent behaviour from one parent to another might well have direct effects such as teaching children aggressive styles of conduct, desensitizing them to violence, distorting their views about conflict resolution, reducing their restraint, and increasing their arousal to aggressive situations. For example, a young mother of two boys who, as a child herself, sat on the stairs at home and listened to her drunken father beat her mother, was referred to an adolescent unit with an eating disorder, and was now living with a partner who beat her. She defended herself with violence, and their violent behaviour was witnessed by her two young boys. She came to therapy because she wanted to stop her violence to her partner and to understand the effect of his violence to her, and her use of violence in self-defence, on her two boys. This was something that had not happened for her as a child, and she was convinced such reflection would be a powerful determinant of her eventual decision. The decision she made was to leave her violent partner.

Suspected physical abuse

If you suspect that a woman may be victimized by her male partner and even assaulted, the priority is to try to assess her safety. You can ask questions with her, either directly or indirectly, depending on the nature of your developing therapeutic alliance. Geffner and Pagelow (1999) identify some helpful questions you might ask when you have the opportunity to meet her on her own, such as:

> Do you feel safer when I talk to you alone?
> Are you afraid of your partner's temper?
> Do you usually give in to stop arguments?
> Are your children afraid when your partner is angry?
> Has your partner ever hit a former partner/his parent(s)/his brothers or sisters/or treated others roughly or disrespectfully?
> Do you feel free to invite neighbours/friends/family to your home?
> Does your partner want to go everywhere with you/listen in on your phone calls/open your mail?
> Is your partner a very jealous person?
> Has your partner threatened to take the children somewhere you cannot find them?
> Does your partner get rough or violent when he's been drinking?
> Has your partner forced you to have sex when you don't want to?
> Have you/your neighbours/your friends ever wanted to call the police because an argument has got out of control?

A priority for safety is to be sure she knows of the existence of her local women's refuge, has the phone number, and the phone number of the local police domestic violence unit. You can enquire if other family members and friends are concerned for her safety and could provide refuge if needed. Ask if she has independent access to money. She may be prepared to meet a police officer and discuss the use of an alarm. Find out if she has a relationship with her family practitioner. Is she able and would she be willing to visit her GP to record visible bruising and other effects of assault? Are there child protection issues that need attention? If social services are involved with the family, ask for permission to liaise with other involved professionals so you can judge the extent of the concern held within the professional system.

In the UK, the coordination of services for victims and perpetrators of domestic violence is done through local domestic violence forums, which often meet quarterly. They provide legislative updates, information on local resources, support for domestic violence policies, and good opportunities to network with other services.

The assessment of risk

In the Reading Safer Families project, Arlene Vetere and Jan Cooper make a distinction between the assessment of risk and the management of risk. If we help with family rehabilitation or do couple's work in the aftermath of violence, it is important to assess for safety first. For example, if we engage in therapeutic work with couples knowing the violence is continuing, we are supporting the violence implicitly at best, and at worst, we are providing the assaulting partner with information about his partner's vulnerabilities.

The assessment of risk is complex. Reder and Lucey (1995), in their book on the assessment of parenting, offer a number of heuristics that can well apply to violence in other family relationships, such as sibling violence, violence of adolescents and young adults towards their parents, violence towards an older person, and violent behaviour from a man to his female partner. These heuristics have been adapted and modified here, using the criteria of systemic therapists who specialize in working with couples where violence is of concern, such as Goldner *et al.* (1990), Jory and Anderson (2000), Vetere and Cooper (2001), and including the work of Jenkins with violent men (1990).

In the assessment of risk, an important distinction is made between *responsibility* for violent behaviour and *explanation* of violent behaviour. Therapeutically and morally, the two are kept separate as there seems to be a cultural tendency to elide the two, as often heard in the linguistic tag, "but I'm not making an excuse" when we offer an explanation for our reprehensible behaviour. Responsibility is assessed by the degree to which a person can acknowledge there is a problem, accept some responsibility for their actions, and recognize that there are relational consequences of their behaviour. When considering family work that involves children, at Reading Safer Families, we do not invite children to family sessions until we have established that parents and carers can develop agency around problem-solving on behalf of their children, particularly in creating a context of safety for their children's future development. Similarly, we do not engage a couple until we have established that the perpetrator of violence can take some responsibility for their behaviour.

We ask questions about repeat violence and the different contexts in which violence has occurred. Clearly if a man, say, is violent in more than one context and has a history of repeat violence, we are less likely to engage in rehabilitative work. We observe carefully his personal boundaries around self-control and anger management, consider whether he has empathy (emotional as well as intellectual) for the experiences of his victim and for his children as witnesses, whether he has the ability to reflect on his past experiences, and whether he can develop internal motivation for change, or whether his motivation is entirely external; for example, court mandated or as a response to his partner's threat to leave him. When talking to parents who have been violent to children, enquiry about their childhood experiences is sometimes met with a blanket response of no recall. Assuming the absence of organic problems and trauma, it is sometimes helpful to reflect systemically on the consequences of not remembering; for example, to whom could the client go for information, what ideas inform his parenting, whom does he look to for ideas about being a father, and so on? We observe whether the person who has been violent consistently blames others for the problems, whether they have respect for social control, and whether they find professional workers potentially helpful to them and their relationships. This is not a checklist, but a guide to assessment of risk and safety. It is unwise to proceed with family work if the family member meets more than a few of the above contra-indications for therapeutic work. However, individual or group work may well provide the context within which some of the contra-indications can be addressed and resolved prior to the initiation of relationally-based work (Vetere and Cooper, 2001, 2003).

When engaging in couple's work, the advice of Jory and Anderson to work quickly to establish an affirming environment for the woman and a challenging environment for the man is helpful. Yet the advice is complex because, at the same time, the therapist needs to establish an empathic relationship with the man, who may well feel shamed and tend to extreme defensiveness as a result. An affirming environment is created by acknowledging a person's right to live without fear in their intimate relationships and by establishing safety, often through the use of a no-violence contract. We shall return to this shortly. A challenging environment can be created by questioning motivation around violence and coming into therapy, helping to develop an awareness of how their actions and attitudes affect their partner and other family members, exploring different ways of thinking and pointing out alternative courses of action, learning about abuse in their family of origin and its relational consequences, and discussing the effects of societal patterns that foster abuse, such as sexism and racism. Recruiting the ghosts of helpful others, living or dead, to whom the violent person can aspire, and helping them to hold the previous generation accountable for their harmful behaviour, are ways that can foster a sense of hopefulness that behaviour can change in the present. Questions that link the past, the present, and the future to the development of patterns and beliefs in families about entitlement to use violence as a strategy of social control, and the ways in which choices have been constrained but might not be so in the future, can be helpful. A genogram can be used to explore patterns of violence in families and those relationships that prove to be exceptions to the problem of violence. Do different beliefs and behavioural choices underpin these different relationships, and if so, how have they been differently constructed and reinforced over time? Are there unspoken rules in the family about who can speak about the violence, about entitlement to use violence, and about who can challenge the violence? An example from the Work of Reading Safer Families illustrates these points. John came to therapy after assaulting his woman partner. He subsequently ended their relationship, partly because he wanted to try to be sure he would not do this again in a future relationship. He was one of three brothers, the eldest of whom beat up their father when they were older adolescents, for beating up their mother over the years, something the brothers had witnessed as children. John told us his father was "good as gold" after that!

The no-violence contract

If rehabilitative work is undertaken with families in the aftermath of violence, it is important to work to establish safety first. This is often effected with the use of a no-violence contract (Carpenter & Treacher, 1989). The perpetrator of violence agrees, either verbally or in writing, to prioritize safety and stop their violent behaviour. The task is to help them achieve this, often using agreed safety strategies, such as time out. Time out is an agreement between the couple that he will take himself to a place of safety, to calm down when aroused, and she will not pursue him or block his exit. If the woman partner also goes to a place of safety, it is important she goes to a part of the house where her exit from the house is not blocked. Men often find physical exercise, such as brisk walking or a work-out, will help reduce tension in the short term and provide some relief. They should be discouraged from use of a vehicle when highly aroused.

When establishing safety strategies, it is important to understand well what the possible triggers for violent behaviour might be. It is helpful to identify the last or the worst episode of violent behaviour as a way of unpicking and understanding the distal and proximal factors that lead to an escalation of conflict into physical violence. In particular, using methods of adapted cognitive behaviour therapy for anger management (Novaco, 1975), make links between self-talk, physiological arousal and perceptions of the partner's intent and behaviour. It is not uncommon to find that men who are violent, and believe they are entitled to use violence to control a woman's behaviour, are more likely to make negative attributions of her behaviour and motivation (Holtzworth-Munroe & Hutchinson, 1993). Using this information, you can problem-solve with the man by using questions such as:

(a) can he identify potential points of conflict and act to de-escalate the interaction?
(b) can he identify his own processes of self talk and physiological arousal and call time out to prevent an escalation into violence?
(c) can his partner agree to the use of the time out strategy?

It is essential that his partner agrees to the use of time out as a way of taking responsibility for her safety and looking after herself. If she pursues him to continue the argument, or blocks his exit, perhaps in the belief that he is using time out to avoid dealing with issues between them, she risks a further escalation of the conflict. She needs to agree to let him go to a place of safety to cool off, and then decide whether they come back to the issue between them or perhaps leave it for discussion at your next meeting. This is often wise in the initial stages of setting up a no-violence contract as it helps to psychologically "safety-net" their attempts to use time out. In addition, always rehearse the use of time out with them both first. Try to predict with them what will get in the way of their use of time out and help them problem-solve a repertoire of responses to situations they can predict are likely to arise between them.

Once the no-violence contract has been established and they have fine-tuned their use of safety strategies with you, you can develop the contract further to include intimidatory behaviour and behaviours designed to denigrate or humiliate the other, such as name-calling. This will form the basis of therapeutic work which addresses wider issues of (a) their parenting and their responsibility for the safety and future well-being of their children; (b) issues of accountability in extended family relationships, particularly if ill-treatment was part of their own experience of growing up; and (c) the legacy of childhood experiences for later beliefs, adult and child attachments, and their own well-being.

Taking women's violence seriously

One of the most difficult challenges for us in our work at Reading Safer Families, was to take women's violence to their male partners seriously (Motz, 2001). When a woman is violent to her child, we have local child protection procedures and The Children Act as a fairly well established frame within which we work. But women's violence to men poses different challenges. For a while it was difficult to address publicly because most of our professional energy went into identifying men's violence to women as the main problem, underpinned by male values of entitlement. Arguably, there is now widespread recognition of the extent of the problem of men's violence to women and, in particular, recognition of the pervasiveness of "patriarchal terrorism", as the Duluth project (Domestic Abuse Intervention Project, 1987) would describe it. This violence is almost exclusively male to female and is more severe. Such public and professional recognition of the problem of men's violence provides a context within which we can now explore the motivations for and effects of women's violence towards their male partners.

The demographic research seems to be in agreement that when women kill their men partners, it is usually in self-defence and often in the context of repeated battering of the woman by the man (Saunders, 1986). Demographic research also shows relatively high rates of violence from women to men, but registers differences in the severity and frequency of attacks, with the general conclusion that, on the whole, women's violence is less hurtful and often not taken seriously by the men themselves. Johnson (1995) has classified this as "common couple violence", i.e. the non-gendered, intermittent response to life's daily frustrations and conflicts. This violence does not form part of a pattern in which the male partner is trying to exert power and control over the woman partner, which is always accompanied by psychological abuse. Women's violence is often in self-defence or is an expression of frustration, stress, and distress, and less often an attempt to control or dominate a partner (James, 1996). Thus, James encourages therapists to differentiate between women who are violent towards an abusive partner and those whose partners are not abusive to them.

We would argue that we do need to take all forms of violence seriously, because of the effects on the victims, the perpetrators, and the children living in violent households. In our clinical experience, the man sometimes hears our concern as an affront to his sense of his masculinity, i.e., a "real" man would not take women's violence seriously. We find at these moments that a careful exploration of what the children are learning in this context, and what the parents would rather the children were learning, using future-oriented questions, helps to overcome embarrassment and the desire to minimize women's violence. Equally, a woman might have behaved in a verbally abusive way as part of a self-defence strategy in the face of her male partner's violence to her, for example, humiliating him, and name-calling. Once the violence has ceased, she may be reluctant to give up her verbally abusive behaviour, feeling entitled to continue having gained the moral high ground as the victim of his violence.

Working in the territory

Psychologists and others who work with people who are assaultative and who have been assaulted listen on an almost daily basis to terrible stories. This is not to underestimate the power of personal accounts of resilience, of hopefulness and resourcefulness, of recovery from harm, and changed attitudes and beliefs around entitlement to hit others. However, our field is currently taken up with stories of survival and resilient behaviour and this possibly makes it harder for us to acknowledge the effects on us of listening to some terrible accounts of intimidation, fear, and harm. Secondary traumatization, as it is called, is serious and should be taken seriously. In passing, we would note the somewhat odd use of the term "secondary", as if it is not primarily distressing at times to listen to such stories and care about what is happening to people. This mirrors the use of the term "witnessing" in the context of the effects on children, which implies an almost neutral watching position for the children! We would suggest regular supervision and consultation to help process the emotional effects of this work and the sources of transference and counter-transference in the work, alongside paying deliberate attention to the sources of your own sustenance, such as other activities and relationships. Where possible, with more worrying cases try to recruit a colleague to work alongside you, either as a co-therapist or in-room consultant (Vetere and Cooper, 2003). Such conjoint activity can help foster a culture of concern that makes contextual changes more possible, such as writing domestic violence policies for your service. Familiarity with the research literature, in our experience, has a helpful preventive effect, by connecting you to a community of like-minded colleagues and keeping you well informed. And finally, pay attention to your own personal safety. Do not work alone in a building, have an alarm in your room, do not sit in such a way that you block access to the door if someone wants to leave quickly, and do not have objects in your room that can be used easily as weapons.

Working with drinking problems

One of us has commented elsewhere that we think systemic approaches have been slow to be adopted within mainstream alcohol treatment approaches, and that the uptake of systemic ideas has been patchy, perhaps reflecting the pattern of uptake of systemic practices across adult mental health settings (Vetere & Henley, 2001). Family systems thinking and therapy can make a helpful contribution to an integrated package of care within a community alcohol service, or can highlight issues when working in other settings where it becomes evident that a family member has a problem with drinking. In addition, systemic ideas integrate well with the Prochaska and DiClemente (1992) model of the stages of change in giving up addictive behaviour, popular within UK-based community alcohol services.

Long-standing problems with drinking can have profound and complex effects on couple relationships and family groups. Orford and Harwin (1982), Velleman (1992) and Velleman *et al.*, (1998) have written in detail about these effects. They include disruption to family members' roles, routines, and communications, disruption to family celebrations, and adverse effects on social life and family finances. For example, there may be difficulties for children in bringing friends home, or being collected safely from school, when a parent is drinking; family celebrations may be spoiled by drunken behaviour; opportunities for socializing may be constrained because of shame and embarrassment; increased risks exist for violent behaviour during arguments; reallocation of family roles may be necessary when a parent is unable reliably to carry out tasks, with the concomitant shifts in power and responsibility and the potential to burden children. The pattern of drinking might result in periods of sobriety and periods of drinking, and for some families the drinking has become the central organizing feature of family life. Thus, when addressing the effects of problem drinking, it is helpful to see family members not only as the context for understanding the problem drinker, but in their own right as possibly in need of a service. For example, understanding the nature of the attachments between couples where drink is a problem is crucial, especially where these attachments are characterized by coercion, violence, and emotional abuse and underpinned by the covert and overt misuse of power; or understanding the repeated patterns of behaviour that may maintain problematic drinking cycles. Systemic psychotherapy provides an overarching framework, with its emphasis on pattern, process, and connection, to help in formulating the nature of the difficulties and planning around change in drinking habits.

Edwards and Steinglass (1995) have summarized the treatment efficacy of twenty-one studies of family involved treatment for drinking problems. Their review concluded: (a) that family involved treatment was marginally more effective than individual treatment; (b) that family therapy helps motivate people with drinking problems into treatment programmes; and (c) that family involved treatment has moderate benefits for relapse prevention.

The findings suggest that three factors mediate the effects of treatment: male gender, family members' continued investment in their relationships, and support from the non-drinking partner for abstinence as a goal. An important caveat for these outcome studies is that they have not included women as the one with the drinking problem, nor have they included the more complex cases. Kent (1990) observed that a man's heavy drinking is more likely to be tolerated by his family and friends over a longer period of time than is a woman's. She observed also that a man is more likely to end his relationship with a woman partner who drinks than is a woman, who is more likely to stay with a heavy-drinking man. However, a woman may well be in a less empowered position both financially and interpersonally, so that her choices for action are different, particularly if she carries the responsibility for the children (Vetere, 1998).

The stages of change

Prochaska and DiClemente (1992) developed the stages of change model, where they suggest that people who try to change habitual behaviour iterate through a series of five stages. Their work has formed the basis of motivational interviewing and contributed to the development of the solution-focused approaches discussed in earlier chapters. The five stages of change are described as follows.

1. Precontemplation—there is no intention to change in the foreseeable future.

2. Contemplation—the person is aware that a problem exists and is thinking about making a change, but has not made the commitment to do so.
3. Preparation—the person intends to take action within the next month and may have already taken some small behavioural steps towards changing.
4. Action—the person changes their problematic behaviour.
5. Maintenance—the person works to prevent relapse and to consolidate what they have achieved.

Relapse is often the rule rather than the exception, in that people often make several attempts to change their behaviour. Prochaska and DiClemente see their model as a spiral, in that some people may well progress through contemplation, preparation, and action, but most will relapse and return to earlier stages in the model. Some may return to pre-contemplation and give up any hope of changing. However, the spiral model suggests that people do not endlessly go round in circles, but rather that each time they relapse, they have an opportunity to learn from their efforts and mistakes and to try to approach things differently next time. Thus, the need to assess a person's readiness to change and tailor interventions accordingly is apparent.

Engagement and consultation

Engagement in couples and family work can be lengthy. The partner with the drinking problem may have developed a primary attachment to alcohol (Vetere & Henley, 2001). The drinker becomes preoccupied with the need to obtain alcohol and all else becomes secondary to this need. Relationships and relationship-maintaining skills may deteriorate because of the lengths to which the drinker will go to maintain a supply of alcohol. Thus, the relationship with an alcohol worker in a community alcohol service, or with a family worker in another service, may be the first significant relationship the drinker has made since alcohol took a hold. Hence, coming into therapy is testing—it may highlight the less-than-optimum relationships in the family and it involves the need to form new relationships.

The commitment to change needs to be prioritized over the commitment to alcohol. Systemic consultation processes can facilitate engagement by providing an opportunity to track the implications of working therapeutically. This careful tracking allows consideration of the differences in motivation for change in the family members' relationships and in their attitudes and responses to issues of blame and responsibility around the problem drinking. Consultation meetings provide early opportunities to externalize the problem with drink and to track the effects on relationships of drinking, while assessing the personal and relationship resources that can be harnessed to combat the effects of problem drinking on relationships.

Reflecting processes

In Chapter Five we examined the use of reflecting processes. Here we shall briefly describe the benefits of reflecting processes when working collaboratively in the room with couples and families, using the model of in-room consultation.

Many of the couples and families seen in a community alcohol service context have been subject to professional scrutiny over long periods of time and the use of a one-way screen might elicit negative transference and interfere with therapeutic engagement. Sometimes, family members can offer harsh, distorting mirrors to their family member who drinks; reflecting processes can offer a kinder, gentler reflection to all as part of the process of recovery and reparation. Systemic reframing can help to identify positive motivation and concern among family members in this context, but not, of course, to reframe responsibility for drinking or abuse. Reflecting conversations can be used to highlight what is going well, to introduce challenging ideas in a non-confrontational way, and to help predict and understand the consequences of a relapse for everyone involved. The invitation to family members to comment and reflect on the therapist–consultant's reflections is a way of privileging their own comments and observations that promotes collaborative practice. The family and small reflecting team provide a container for processing strong emotions and together create a context for the use of systemic reframing, which encompasses the norms and practices of the larger society in which we live.

Pattern and process in relationships

Systemic thinking and practice is part of a multi-modal approach to working with individuals and their families where long-standing patterns of drinking dominate family life. The intersect between patterns of drinking and patterns in family relationships over time provides a focus for the exploration of family culture, beliefs, and life-cycle transitions (Vetere & Henley, 2002).

1. Pattern in communication

The task for therapy is to develop honest and straight talking about the drinking. Accusations of lying from the non-drinking partner, about whether the person has been drinking, or whether they have hidden bottles of alcohol about the house and garden, or even whether they have attended their appointments, often abound. The drinking partner may well feel shamed or be shamed by their non-drinking partner. One of the longer-term effects of problem drinking is to limit communication, and this leads to the withholding of intimate information, constricting exchange and communication in the partnership. Feelings of shame and humiliation act as a barrier to the development of openness and honesty in conversation and to rebuilding trust in the relationship. Alcohol may represent an escape from intolerable feelings and can become entrenched as an over-learned pattern of coping, with different meanings ascribed to the drinking by different family members. For the non-drinking partner, there is often a struggle to trust that drinking will not begin again. This is where systemic reflecting processes can be so helpful in raising and addressing these issues in a non-blaming way.

If the non-drinking partner has taken a position on the moral high ground from where they shame and humiliate their drinking partner about the effects of their drinking, the patterns and expectancies around behaviour can be harder to deconstruct. The legacy of shame and contempt from the non-drinking partner can persist while the drinking partner revolves around the stages of change, seemingly unable to change and reinforcing the idea they are unable to accept responsibility for their behaviour. In these circumstances, it seems to us that the non-drinking partner holds a belief that they do not need to change, almost as if they are in the pre-contemplation stage of change. However, if change does occur, sometimes couples move to contemplate separation as they address the long tern legacy of shame and contempt in their relationship.

2. Pattern in relationships

Over time, couple relationships may have fallen into patterns of complementarity, where one partner dominates and power is not held equitably, or into symmetry, where both partners compete for power, such as, who knows best, or has the last word, or whose view of reality prevails. The lack of felt satisfaction in the relationship and the lack of psychological rewards can be discomfiting and differently acknowledged. The drinking partner, for example, may well continue their pattern of drinking to escape or avoid such discomfort. The non-drinking partner may then use this as evidence that change is unlikely, or to bolster their view that the problem lies with the drinking partner. The effects of living in complementary or symmetrical relationships can vary according to whether the drinker is a man or a woman. For a woman in a complementary relationship, her drinking may be seen as evidence of her incompetence or contemptibility, which may reinforce her sense of powerlessness and inability to effect change for herself. However, her attempts to assert her point of view can be seen as aggression and further used against her, reinforcing patterns of blame. Paradoxically, her male partner may well feel helpless, distressed, and frustrated about his ability to change her behaviour. This could pose a risk of abuse.

It is helpful to listen to couples' descriptions of behaviour, attitudes, decision-making, and styles of conflict resolution, in order to understand how they share power in their relationship. When talking about drinking and its effects, we can hear descriptions of feeling powerful and feeling powerless. Asking to what extent access to power is gendered, and whether resources have changed over time, or at different life-cycle stages, with adaptation to drinking or to stopping drinking, paves the way to talking about personal responsibility and developing a sense of personal agency, for both drinking behaviour and the responses to drinking behaviour.

If the drinker's primary relationship with alcohol shifts into the action and maintenance stages of change, there are systemic consequences for all family members. People are sometimes unprepared for the impact that stopping drinking has on their relationships. For example, other methods of coping are not always easily developed by the drinking partner, and for the non-drinking partner, used to uncovering evidence of drinking with the skills of a detective, it can be hard to give up this behaviour. Couples often find they need to reassess the basis of their relationship, and they do this when the drinker is in the maintenance stage of change. When the view of the future is filled with anticipated loss and lack of direction, "future" questions can be helpful in exploring contrasting views of the future in which drinking continues and does not continue (Penn, 1985). Imagining a future without drinking, in a solution-focused way (Miller & Berg, 1995), encourages people to reflect on aspects of family life organized in response to the problem drinking. When working with women as the problem drinkers, we have noticed that when she becomes more independent, her male partner agrees to work towards a more reciprocal relationship, thus shedding some of the patterns of complementarity.

3. Patterns over time

We talk to couples and family members about their understanding of life-cycle demands. Curiosity about "why now?" in response to a request for consultation can develop discussion about changing life-cycle demands and aspirations. For example, a wife who drank throughout her husband's career may find retirement poses different challenges and long-term plans have to be shelved because of her drinking. Alternatively, his drinking may lead to unplanned early retirement, perhaps at a time when they have increased financial responsibilities for adolescent children. It is this exploration of the intersect between problem drinking and life-cycle demands, for all family members, that provides the opportunity to understand how family life has revolved around the problem drinking. They may have become a problem-determined system (Anderson *et al.*, 1986), with family members trying to deny or minimize the effects of drinking, trying to protect others from the effects of the drinking, or trying to ostracize the drinker. These patterns of behaviour can become reinforced and entrenched over time. The crisis that precipitates a move into therapeutic work provides the opportunity to unpack these patterns in a non-blaming way, with opportunities to reframe people's behaviour as capable of change. Recruiting supportive and positive figures from the family's past can help when exploring distressing and shameful memories.

In conclusion, couples and family work can be demanding, both because of the marked power imbalances in relationships and the lack of intimate communication, whereby drinking has come between them. For example, couples may well be fearful that any communication will make an already tense situation worse. In our experience, therapeutic progress depends both on the drinking partner being able to re-establish relationships within the family, where the relationship with alcohol is no longer primary, and on the non-drinking partner acknowledging that they, too, need to change. Stopping drinking does not always bring the happiness so long desired.

Working with eating disorders

Eating disorders are arguably one of the most intractable and deadly of the psychiatric disorders. In the case of anorexia the rate of mortality is reported to be around 20% (Bryant-Waugh & Lask, 1995). Bulimia can lead to severe problems induced by continual vomiting leading to serious medical problems. Likewise, obesity can lead to serious medical problems such as heart failure. Apart from these obvious medical problems all the conditions are associated with social isolation, withdrawal, low self-esteem and, in many instances, depression. Treatments for all three conditions are also notoriously difficult (Fairburn *et al.*, 2002). There is no clearly established treatment that has a convincingly high rate of success, which in part has prompted the move into the multi-modal treatments that are now popular. Possibly this is one of the reasons that attempts to offer a treatment for eating disorders has played such a significant part in the development of family therapy. In effect, family therapy was often the last hope for many families that contained a member suffering from these debilitating disorders.

Attempts to offer a treatment for eating disorders, especially anorexia, has featured prominently in the history of family therapy. Returning to our three phases of family therapy outlined in Chapter One we can see that each phase had at least one major attempt at approaching the treatment of eating disorders:

1. **Structural**—Minuchin and his colleagues (1978) suggested that anorexia could be seen as evolving in a particular family context

that encouraged the development of psychosomatic symptoms. The ingredients of such family contexts he suggested were:

- A pattern of conflict avoidance
- Weak parental executive—inability of the parents to work together in making decisions for their children's well-being
- Enmeshment or over-involvement between one or both parents and the child
- Triangulation—the child's symptoms as functioning to regulate or detour the conflict between the parents. Typically, this conflict was seen as covert and only expressed through disagreements about how to deal with the child's eating disorders.

2. **Systemic**—In the second phase of family therapy, the ideas of the Milan school figured highly in work with families with anorexia (Selvini-Palazzoli, 1974). In some ways, although advocating quite a different philosophy underlying the treatment, they shared some of the observations regarding the family dynamics underlying anorexia described above. For example, while advocating an approach that was much less concerned with attempting to generate normative descriptions about family dynamics, they nevertheless commented that the disorder seemed to be associated with some common family features, such as an apparent "niceness" and lack of any conflict. Likewise, they also noted what they described as the marital "stalemate"—a moribund marital relationship in which conflicts and dissatisfactions had gone underground. In contrast to the structural approaches, the Milan therapists emphasized that the underlying, and typically covert, beliefs were central to an understanding of anorexia. In particular, they suggested that a central part of the beliefs was that feelings were dangerous and should not be expressed. Furthermore, they noted that in many of the families there had been a transition from a relatively rural lifestyle to a smarter urban life in which appearance, slimness, and beauty carried a much greater premium. The mothers of young people suffering with anorexia were seen as caught between these two lifestyles and their daughters were covertly expressing this conflict. The Milan therapists argued that the fathers in these families wanted their wives to be both "modern" women and safe and domesticated. They went on to suggest that the mothers experienced competing

pressures, perhaps with their own mothers expecting them to be traditional mothers but modern urban society making them feel out of place if they did conform to the traditional role. These generational and societal pressures encouraged tensions within a marriage and could lead to conflicts in which the daughters could become embroiled. More specifically, again in some agreement with the structural approaches, the Milan school suggested that patterns of secret coalitions could develop so that the daughter with anorexia was particularly singled out to take sides with each parent against the other. The reasons why one child might be singled out could include the particular dynamics of the family at that time, her physical appearance, and/ or the history of the relationship with each parent.

3. **Narrative approaches**. Although the third phase of family therapy is less characterized by distinct approaches and techniques, a number of themes can be seen in relation to work with eating disorders and families. In particular, there has been more emphasis on recognizing the social context; for example, that extent to which ideas of beauty and body image are central aspects of female identity, especially in relatively affluent Western cultures. This has prompted an approach to work with families that is less exclusively focused on the internal family dynamics and pays attention to how broader conflicts around gender—such as power and inequality—are played out in the domain of family life. Michael White (1987), has posited that young women with anorexia may be caught up in a contradictory position of loyalty to traditional values of femininity and domesticity but at the same time influenced by modern, feminist critiques of this position. As an illustration, he points to the frequently observed phenomenon that many young women with anorexia make considerable attempts to produce food for their family that they will not eat themselves. In a sense this can be seen as a sort of tragic parody of the conventional domestic role—the nurturing and self-sacrificing mother. We can see that this analysis connects with some of the earlier observations of Selvini-Palazzoli (1974). This fits with the broader observation that typically these young women have been seen as "good" girls who never overtly rebelled in any way, usually achieving highly academically and in most ways being "perfect" young women. The onset of anorexia can

be seen to signal a change in this conformity, although this is rarely expressed overtly as rebellion but more as an attack on the self. Bruch (1978) and others have described this as anger turned against the self. Interestingly, mothers and daughters can be seen to be caught in a struggle that is not of their own making but is due to the influence of cultural values. For example, in our clinical experience we have observed that the mothers typically disagree with the suggestion that the anorexia is in some ways caused by the social pressures on women to be slim and beautiful. Instead, they appear to be caught in perpetuating or implementing these oppressive ideas and practices with their own daughters. Possibly to resist these might require a painful examination of the extent to which they themselves have been coerced to accept their domestic and societal duties.

A large part of the focus in families has been on the role of the mother–daughter relationship but increasingly there is interest in the role of fathers. We have observed in our clinical work and research that frequently fathers appear to be closely, and at times uncomfortably, involved with the young women; for example, having knowledge of their daughters' bodies, menstruation, physical state, eating and sleeping patterns. This over-involvement seems at the same time to be regulated by some emotional distance, even a covert hostility, between the daughter and her mother. In a sense, a theme appears to be that the daughter in some ways is positioned as representing the wife the husband would like his actual wife to be—slim, beautiful, and yet a good, dutiful, domesticated woman. The mother's resentment at this role may then be seen to be directed at her daughter, who is held up as being able to carry off this contradictory representation. Underlying this there also appears to be a pattern of emotional and sexual distance in the marriage (Selvini-Palazzoli, 1974; Bruch, 1978). This can be a dangerous position for the daughter, and one way to avoid becoming an object of her father's frustrated desires is to remain a pretty, non-sexual little girl. One sure way of achieving this is to starve oneself so that sexual development is delayed. One of us (AV) has twice worked with families where, apparently without the mothers' knowledge, the fathers asked the daughters to dress for them, in secret, in their mothers' clothing. A related example is where a young girl had discussed with her father her intentions to live with him in the event of the parents separating.

In contemporary practice the distinctions between these approaches in clinical work with eating disorders is less clear. For example, most approaches assume that a central component of the work, especially with younger people, is to facilitate the ability of the parents to be able to work together to encourage the young person to return to a safe weight. This can essentially be a structural approach that aims at strengthening the parents' ability or power to take care of their child's physical well-being. This orientation can be complemented by ideas from narrative therapy; for example, the idea of "externalizing" the anorexia and exploring how the family members together can resist the effects it is having on the young person and support her in resisting the eating disorders. Often this also involves an eventual focus on the nature of the marital relationship. For example, in one current case (RD) the sessions have moved to couples work with the parents that is exploring the viability of the marriage, and a central component of this has been the nature of the couple's sexual relationship (Figure 2). Where the parents are able to reflect on their own dynamics in a relatively open way, this appears to be associated with better outcome than where the apparent conflicts and tensions remain covert (Dallos & Hamilton Brown, 2000; Selvini-Palazzoli, 1974).

Most eating disorders services also offer considerable individual input to the person showing the eating disorder. This can be of the

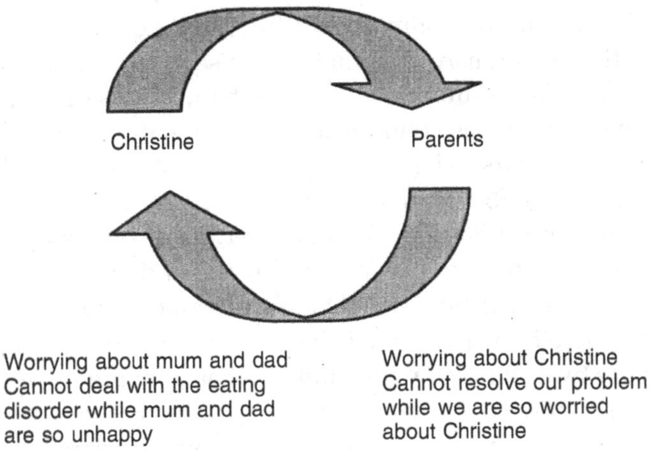

Figure 2. A "worrying" cycle: Being unable to deal with one's own problems while worrying about those of others.

kind of individual systemic work described by Boscolo and Bertrando (1996), but often it typically involves approaches such as CBT, CAT or psychodynamic work. It is important that this therapeutic work is considered within a wider systemic framework, so that, for example, the emphasis does not simply shift to a view of the problems as simply residing in the person showing the eating disorder. As with many forms of therapeutic work, it is essential to consider the timing and relationships between the different types of therapeutic input. In the case described above the parents only felt able to work on their own issues in the context of knowing that their daughter was relatively safe in respect of her health and had formed a good working relationship with an individual therapist. In turn, it was clear that she was more able to benefit from her individual work as she became more reassured that her parents were getting some help and she no longer felt that she needed to carry the full burden of responsibility for worrying about her parents.

This multiple approach also recognizes that although the analysis of family and cultural dynamics may be compelling, it is also clear that the physiological changes triggered by self-starvation produce, among other things, hormonal changes which are then resistant to reversal. In effect, a form of illness does result, and even if the family dynamics alter the biological processes, they may need treatment and time to be reversed.

A focus on the marital dynamics can appear to suggest a blaming perspective. However, in our work we encourage an exploration of the traditions of attachment across the generations. For example, there is increasing evidence that there is a trans-generational tradition of insecure and predominantly avoidant or dismissive attachment styles (Feeney & Noller, 1996). This involves a culture of emotional avoidance and difficulties in dealing with conflicts, relationships and feelings. The core marital dynamic in the family may be shaped by the styles of relating that have been learned in the parents' own childhoods (Dallos, 2001).

Working with families in services for people with learning disabilities

Hatton *et al.*, (1999) recently edited a special feature on learning disabilities for *The Psychologist*. In an article making the case for inclusion, they pointed out that demographic changes indicated that people with learning difficulties were living longer, that children with complex and very severe needs were surviving into adulthood, and, most importantly, they carry a higher risk of developing mental health problems than the general population. The past twenty years have seen the effects of a major policy shift with the closure of the segregated hospitals and the advent of community care, which in many cases means family-based care. New patterns of migration and acculturation in families need to be reflected in policy, planning, and service development. Psychologists have much to offer in helping change people's lives for the better. The main thrust of this section is to examine the claim that systemic ideas and practice can be influential in meeting the challenges and opportunities posed by care in the community.

Systemic ideas have taken longer to develop in services for people with learning disabilities, for a number of reasons that one of us has bemoaned elsewhere (Vetere, 1996). Latterly, however, there seems to be a shift in the professional consensus towards the inclusion of systemic ideas and practices, perhaps influenced by users' groups, the disability and human rights movements, policy and recent legislation, and the increasing number of models of stress and coping. The family systems approaches would both (a) posit that social and environmental factors are crucial in their effects on families with members with learning disabilities, and (b) help us map the complex professional networks within which these families live their lives.

Sloper (1999) identified some families who continue to have high levels of unmet needs: (a) those with more than one disabled child; (b) some ethnic minority families; (c) parents with older children; and (d) families where there is severe impairment. User surveys have highlighted persistently that family carers ask for services to give them information and advice on how to help their child, to offer respite services, and other practical support, and a key-worker model whose main task is to help them negotiate their way through complex professional systems (Beresford, 1994). The features of effective help-giving have been summarized in the work of Dunst and colleagues (1994) to be characterized by: (a) open and honest communication; (b) an emphasis on relationship-building with family members; (c) understanding the parents and family members' own appraisals and concerns; and (d) responsiveness to family values, goals and aspirations. These ideas fit well with systemic practice.

There is a growing body of empirical evidence to support the effectiveness of the family and marital therapies, across a range of ages, developmental needs, and service areas (Carr, 2000a,b). Stenfert-Kroese *et al.*, (1997), when writing of the effectiveness of cognitive behaviour therapies for adults with learning disabilities, argue that it is more appropriate to adapt existing models and practices than to develop an entirely separate evidence base. We support this position, in that emotional and attachment needs across the family life-cycle are higher-order constructs for our work, with specific reference paid to family members' needs on a case by case basis.

In thinking about the usefulness of systemic ideas and practice within this service, a number of significant issues provide a framework for working with families and complex networks, as detailed below.

1. Convene the network of concern, including the extended family

Families who care for children and adults with disabilities are sometimes characterized by shrinking social networks. For example, concerns about others' reactions to a child's behaviour or appearance might, over a period of time, lead to less social activity, difficulty in finding substitute carers, and fewer friends for the couples. Thus, careful consideration of who is out there for the family, where they obtain their support, both emotional and social, and whether we might have a role in helping to expand contracted networks, are important systemic considerations.

Alternatively, while the family's social network may shrink, their professional network often expands at an exponential rate! Martin's (1989) survey found that families might be involved with between ten and twenty of the forty different identified professions at any one time. The task for parents and carers in managing the boundaries of shared responsibilities, decision-making, and information sharing with professionals is always complex and not without its tensions. For example, a family raising children might find themselves dealing with multiple outsiders and sharing decisions over one child, but not for the other children in the family, and this may well continue into their adulthood. Any request for our involvement should always be followed by a mapping of the network of concern, showing clearly who is already involved with the family and why, what the history of liaison has been, and what mechanisms exist for dealing with any differences and disagreements over the care of the child. The potential for the boundary to blur between parental and agency responsibility for decision-making around the child or adult can be complicated further by the well documented tendency for parents to air their anxieties about their child with whichever professional worker they have developed the closest relationship (Martin, 1989). (Working with complex networks is, of course, discussed more fully in Chapter Five.)

2. Engagement with the family, including fathers

There are no easy answers to the difficulties of sharing power when engaging parents and families. Services on the whole have a commitment to partnership models of service delivery and to ways of working that take account of the diversity between families and between parents and professionals (Dale, 1996). The Children Act recognizes that families have a key role in a child's life and family systems thinking helps identify the complex weave of children's needs and family process and functioning. When mapping the referral system, it is instructive to talk to the family members about their "relationship to help", as described in Chapter Five. Families rarely come fresh to a service. They usually have a history of relationships with our multi-disciplinary colleagues. However, it could be said that some services engage with the primary carer, often the mother addressing correspondence to one parent only, and making assumptions about carers' roles and beliefs as teachers and educators of children. Early intervention schemes may be aimed at the mother as primary carer, and probably do not consider the systemic consequences for her other relationships (e.g., with the father and with siblings) of the possible intensification of the parent–child relationship. If the mother has the main responsibility for meeting the many professionals involved in her child's care, she has many opportunities to confide and process her feelings of grief that may not be available to the other parent, with longer-term consequences for their differential adaptation and adjustment to looking after a child with disabilities.

Convening fathers takes on a different importance in the light of these comments. Very little research has explored fathers' roles in the care of their children with disabilities (Lamb & Billings, 1997). The research that exists presents us with an inconsistent picture: we know little about how fathers spend their time with their children and how much of their time, or how they and their relationships are affected by raising a child with disabilities. Most studies have focused on fathers' reactions to receiving a diagnosis of disability and to their initial adaptation. Overall, if their main role in the family is to work in outside employment, their stress levels are reported to be lower, but so is their satisfaction with family life, compared with that of other fathers who are more involved in caring for their children. They report sensitivity to social norms. Active involvement in planning around the child's needs, combined with high levels of social support, can contribute to the further development of personal values and personal growth. Recent work by Walters *et al.* (2001) would suggest that fathers' regular attendance at family therapy meetings in children's services might be predicted by their positive experiences with their own fathers and by high levels of satisfaction in their relationship with their partner. The implications are clear. If we do not actively convene fathers and offer our services at times they can attend, we risk ignoring fathers' emotional needs and their actual and potential roles in families.

We might be at risk of under-focusing the role of siblings in our work with families. Goodyer (1990) notes that, in his experience, parents often do not want to include siblings in the therapy. Yet, brothers and sisters can be very involved in the care of a disabled sibling, often with the effect of reversing expected chronological roles. Research findings are equivocal when tracking the effects of these role changes over time. Some researchers write of the benefits for siblings of increased parental expectations and of developing compassion and social competence, while others write of longer-term psychological costs to emotional well-being (Gath & Gumley, 1987).

It is important to note that some parents need help to secure practical support such as respite facilities and aids, adaptations, and welfare benefits before they are ready to work on behavioural problems or their emotional concerns (Smale, 1978). Although this may not be our direct task, as members of complex professional networks we are often in a position to facilitate liaison and information, so that subsequent engagement in our service may be facilitated.

3. The importance of family life-cycle stages

Family life-cycle theories (Carter & McGoldrick, 1989) remind us that any individual, at any time in their lives, can be thought of as nested within a complex and fluid three- to four-generational system of relationships. Thus, people are, so to speak, looking up the system, down the system, and within their own generation to find meaning in their experiences and to live out their extended family relationships. Individuals without family to speak of, may still find themselves subject to others' normative beliefs about what they might be expected to be doing at any point in their lives, and this social comparison combined with their own expectations may help shape their responses to life-cycle transitions. Lynggaard *et al.*, (2001) write about the value of systemic approaches in working with residential staff and multi-disciplinary teams. (See Chapter Two for a more detailed description of the family life-cycle approach.)

Family life-cycle theories also remind us that times of transition, both expected and unexpected and untimely, along with expansion and contraction of the system, are likely to be more stressful because they make demands on our coping and challenge our beliefs about predictability. For families raising children with disabilities and caring for adults, life-cycle transitions may not occur when chronologically expected, or not at all, in some instances, requiring further and different adjustments. Systemic approaches to practice can be helpful to families at different times in their own family development. Some of the difficulties that may occur are:

- educational statementing procedures and the requirement that parents be explicit about their child's abilities;
- issues of social comparison and social isolation for the young adolescent in terms of their own developing sense of autonomy;
- the transition of leaving home for many may be psychologically marked by independent employment and establishing one's own intimate relationships and family life—this is sometimes less possible for young adults with disabilities and sexuality is seen more as a risk than as a human need and right;

- whether or not to ask for genetic counselling in the light of heritable conditions;
- decisions about respite and future placement if the caring adult becomes unable to continue with the task;
- changing relationships with siblings over the life-cycle;
- forming relationships with changing professional staff.

4. Themes of loss and coping

It is curious that we know more about loss and grief in families who care for someone with disabilities than we do about their strengths, coping, and resources. Perhaps this reflects earlier beliefs, now discredited, that families with members with disabilities were "handicapped families" (Tew, 1974). Since the middle of the 1980s the literature has moved to a stress and coping perspective, which recognizes both a diversity in family members' responses and that material, personal, and social resources relate to parental well-being (Folkman & Lazarus, 1980). The approach taken in this book assumes that parental distress is not inevitable, but where it does occur, particularly in a context of poor social support, it is to be taken seriously. This is based on the belief that parental well-being and morale will influence the quality of care given to children and adults for whom they have responsibility. The parents' overall style of problem-solving seems to be important to meeting successfully the challenges of raising a child with disabilities. For example, a constructive and problem-oriented style seems to be more helpful than one where emotional reactions are ignored, or where emotional reactions are experienced and not processed (Beavers *et al.*, 1986). Where there are two parents (or a well supported lone parent), constructive problem-solving includes teamwork, the ability to acknowledge differences of opinion and methods of negotiation, and conflict resolution (*ibid.*).

It has been suggested that experiences of loss and grieving have the potential to be re-evoked at different stages of the family life-cycle as the person with disabilities negotiates expected and unexpected transitions in life along with other family members. For example, parents might be reminded of a child's limitations during the education statementing process, or the balance between protectiveness and personal autonomy might be challenged when the young adult is recommended to live in semi-independent accommodation. Patterns of grieving across the generations may well reflect patterns in relationships. For some family members, inability to acknowledge the extent and range of grief reactions can lead to what has been called "life-cycle freezing" where patterns of coping suitable to a child of a much younger age persist well into adulthood. Alternatively, a chronic sorrow might develop over time, leading to an emotionally flattening effect within intimate interactions, or the inability to accept a diagnosis of disability could lead to "shopping around" for a different diagnosis, which complicates the implementation of procedures of assessment and a package of care (Black, 1987). Strong protective feelings and behaviours can be evoked at times of transition, particularly the transition into adulthood. Since many of the accepted rites of passage are not possible for young adults with moderate and severe disabilities, there are few culturally acceptable markers of changed status. Yet the attempt by the young person to seek a degree of autonomy can sometimes invigorate a protective constraining response, based on fear of danger, risk and loss, and a wish to protect the person from the consequences of their disability. Equally, a protective response might be experienced as a defence against anxiety or guilt when a carer experiences strong feelings of ambivalence about their role or their emotional reactions to their family member. Grief often provides the emotional context for such experiences. These are sensitive issues for interpretation and are often seen in hindsight when piecing together different accounts of a family's history of relationships with services.

5. The importance of rituals and use of non-verbal communication in therapy

The move to narrative and emphasis on discourses within the field of psychotherapy are appraised cautiously in this context, not because people with learning disabilities do not hold narratives about themselves and others, but because there is a risk that verbal interaction is unduly privileged over non-verbal interaction. Therapy with families may need to be more slowly paced and reflective (Goldberg *et al.*, 1995) because the day to day demands of caring may not have left much time for such reflection. Silence needs to be understood for what it is—inability to speak, lack of practice with speaking, or not knowing what to say—in order to prevent "speaking for" or "interpreting for" where it might not be necessary or helpful. These are sensitive issues and the therapist needs to beware taking over the "speaking for" role in this work. In our experience this is more likely when the therapist is more reliant on verbal interaction and is shy of experimenting with non-verbal methods of communication.

A decision needs to be taken about whether and when to include the person with disabilities in the work, depending on their age, their abilities, and their wish to participate (when it is known). If participation is feasible, the therapist may well wish to promote inclusion by adapting practical strategies and play methods appropriate to the age of the client. For example, using drawing, sculpting, role-plays, model-making, cartoon characters, and analogue scales to represent emotional experiences, actions, and events; using enactment rather than verbal descriptions; and using a form of "circular showing" via role-play and enactment to represent circularity and recursiveness in behaviour before exploring understanding through the use of circular questions (Fiddell, 2000; Vetere, 1993).

It is not uncommon to find that children and adults with disabilities are excluded from key cultural rituals such as funerals or weddings. The exclusion is often motivated by a desire to protect from loss, or a belief that the person will not understand and become confused. But such exclusion does not recognize that emotional maturity is not the same as intellectual maturity and loses the opportunity for benefit from a shared cultural experience and meaningful participation for all.

Family therapy

The above framework makes the case for the value of systemic ideas and practice with families with members with learning disabilities. However, from time to time, a family may well benefit from family therapy in the more formal and contractual sense. The rest of this section will consider some of the issues that are brought forward for more focused therapeutic work. The approach advocated here tries to be collaborative, gender and culture sensitive, and, we hope, user-friendly (Reimers, 2001), and acknowledges that the best judges will be the families themselves.

Acceptance of a diagnosis

There is some evidence that a clear diagnosis is helpful to parents (Black, 1987). It can offer a pathway into appropriate services and enable a realistic appraisal of a child and adult's needs and abilities. Such realism is thought to facilitate day to day coping and goals more oriented to the present (Beavers *et al.*, 1986). Where a diagnosis is unavailable or a parent is unable or unwilling to accept a diagnosis, or the more "normal" the child appears to be, there seems to be an elevated risk of relying on denial as an emotional coping mechanism. For example, when working in a child development centre, one of us (AV) would find that physiotherapists and occupational therapists approached her for advice on why an otherwise "intelligent" parent might not follow advice on exercises for the child designed to prevent "windswept" deformity. If the parent/s was willing to meet, it was not uncommon to find that any denial of the nature and implications of the child's condition was underpinned by powerful and unexpressed feelings of grief. Clearly this would have systemic implications for the quality of the couple communication following the diagnosis of their child's condition.

Psychoeducational approaches

Many parents want information and advice on how best to promote their child's development and how to cope with developmental tasks (Sloper, 1989). Quine and Pahl (1989) estimate that over half of children with disabilities experience severe settling and waking problems. These behaviours might continue for many years, and are often associated with difficult daytime behaviour and family-wide stress. In their study of families with children with Downs syndrome, Byrne *et al.*, (1988) found that half the mothers interviewed expressed lasting concerns about the way they had handled their children. As part of a solution, Byrne *et al.*, (1988) suggest that when parents are offered behavioural strategies, they need to understand the principles behind them so that they can design their own plans for action. This helps parents interpret their child's behaviour more accurately and positively. From a systemic point of view, it is important to take account of family dynamics when helping to implement advice and behavioural interventions.

The expression of complex feelings

While giving birth to a child with an identifiable handicapping condition is an enriching experience for some families, for others it is not. It may be appropriate to address issues of emotional unavailability and withdrawal or compensatory over-protection with specific bereavement work, which enables the naming and expression of the unsaid, such as difficult and complex emotions of shame, disgust, anger, and disappointment.

Relating as a family to problems

Living with disability affects everyone in the family group. Beavers *et al.*, (1986), in their research on family coping, suggest that where family life is organized around the needs of one member, rather than differently prioritizing others' needs at different times, there is likely to be decreased satisfaction for other members. Identifying and reflecting on family roles within family subsystems and promoting flexibility of relating and communication is a means of addressing problems with blurred boundaries and rigid or diffuse communication. Family therapy sessions can offer siblings an opportunity to establish their points of view and explore the impact on them of living with a brother or sister with learning disabilities. We have discussed earlier in this section the role of social support networks. Trute and Hauch (1988) found that positive family adaptation to the birth of a child with multiple disabilities was linked to parents' skilful use of family and friendship networks. Their research highlights the need for family therapists to assess the availability of support and to help families mobilize and access their social resources.

Parental teamwork

Arguably, parental health, energy, and morale are intimately linked with the quality of their couple relationship in an iterative process. There would appear to be a relationship between the strength of the couple's adjustment and positive family functioning, regardless of the age of the child, or their level of disability, or the family's income (Beavers *et al.*, 1986; Trute & Hauch, 1988). However, parents can be overtaxed by their child's supervision needs from time to time, and may struggle to differentiate between parental tensions and couple tensions. The ability to disagree as parents, while maintaining a commitment to teamwork, seems to be a helpful position for many parents, and one in which they can maintain a commitment to their couple relationship. The task of the therapist is sometimes to create a reflective space to explore and discuss their options as parents and partners.

In concluding this section, we hope we have shown how systemic ideas can inform intervention and how family therapy can be helpful at particular times in families' lives. Just as family members' needs, resources, and aspirations change over time, so, too, do our services and interventions need to change in response so that we remain flexible and accessible in what we can offer families.

The importance of multi-modal treatment approaches

Some of the interpersonal problems and dilemmas described in the sections above are sufficiently complex in terms of their formulation for clinical practice to benefit from a deliberate attempt to integrate different explanatory frameworks. Additionally, such complexity often benefits from a clinical approach that combines individual work with couples work and a family- and significant relationships-based approach to intervention. Such an approach is flexible and promotes continuous, systematic review of clinical hypotheses and clinical practices in relation to the nature of the interpersonal difficulties. A systemic approach to practice provides a useful umbrella under which to contain such complexity and to review effectiveness. When such a flexible approach explicitly draws together different modalities of psychotherapy and mixes them with individual and family-based work, the approach is sometimes called a multi-modal approach to intervention. It finds its application with the more complex clinical problems, with families with multi-agency relationships, and with families who require Tier Three interventions and Social Services' involvement because of the complex social and psychological needs of the family members.

One of the core competencies that clinical psychologists, amongst others, hope to be able to offer is the ability to employ and evaluate different treatment models. Perhaps more than other clinical groups, clinical psychologists are trained to employ and integrate different theoretical frameworks and their concomitant treatment techniques or styles. Systemic approaches, from their outset, have attempted to be integrative and adapted to offer a trans-theoretical model of how productive change occurs (Watzlawick *et al.*, 1974). As systemic family therapy became established, sometimes this integrative, multi-model base was obscured. However, more recently a commitment to a multi-modal approach, especially in the context of complex problems, has again been explicitly stated.

Pinsof and Wynne, in their 1995 review of the efficacy and effectiveness of the marital and family therapies, noted that there is increasing evidence for the value of treatment packages, of which family therapy is a part, for therapeutic work with families where a member has a diagnosis of schizophrenia (Vaughan & Leff, 1976), or for more severe adolescent conduct disorders and problems with delinquent behaviour. Carr (2000a), in his review, added therapeutic work with children and families where child abuse and neglect are issues, and emotional and psychosomatic problems as benefiting from a multi-modal approach.

For example, the so-called family intervention studies have consistently shown that relapse rates for another episode of psychosis can be reduced by working with families directly on issues of day to day living and coping. Assisting family members to change the emotional climate within the home, or the levels of "expressed emotion" can help reduce the felt experience of stress, which is believed to be linked to heightened risk of onset and relapse in psychosis (Goldstein & Miklowitz, 1995). Importantly, the family intervention studies are often carried out within a package of care that may include anti-psychotic medication and efforts to reduce the amount of face-to-face contact time family members spend with each other. Although studies have attempted to partial out the active ingredients of the treatment package, the way forward seems to lie with integrated treatments that include family work.

From a systemic perspective, the family intervention approaches raise a number of issues that need tackling when used as part of an overall package of care. It is important to emphasize that all family members are offered assistance, and not just seen in the context of a method to aid symptom reduction for the "patient" (Gopfert, personal communication). A family intervention suggests we need to have "joined-up" services and referral strategies which, lamentably, do not exist in most UK Health Trusts. We still come across circumstances in which a parent has been referred to the acute psychiatry service, the partner may be referred to another adult psychotherapy service, and the child may be referred to children's services. Acute adult psychiatry services still do not recognize the "patient" as a parent and engage with their parental concerns, but the adoption of a systemic perspective would aid the understanding of people in their multiple roles and responsibilities and this in turn would have direct consequences for service provision. Thus, the phenomenon of "intermittent parenting" caused by in-patient admissions or periods of acute distress could be understood in a way that would help people plan and deal with it. Another example rests in the finding that late adolescence is a period for the onset of a psychosis. Systemically speaking, late adolescence is a period of transition within both the individual and the family life-cycle; therefore, any service for older adolescents and young adults will have a direct impact on these life-cycle changes and adaptations.

Reaping the benefits from the family intervention studies by implementing family-based services presupposes that practitioners are skilled in establishing working alliances with family members. User and carer surveys often show that family members want to be seen as part of the solution, not as part of the problem, but are often ignored (Prior, personal communication). Most practitioners are trained to work with individuals, to see the "psychosis" as the problem, and to work in systems and organizations that promote individual work. It is of interest to note that the National Service Framework clearly sees the psychological therapies as part of long-term care and states that the family members of those who have serious mental health difficulties should have an assessment of their needs and a written care plan. Fadden (1998) observes that many clinicians find it difficult to work with families and lack confidence in their abilities to establish positive alliances. Training alone does not always seem to help. The system as a whole needs to be influenced. It may be that clinical governance will help, as at all Trust levels some standards for the psychological therapies, including family intervention, will need to be stated.

Burbach and Stanbridge (1998) provide an interesting and tested example of a family-based approach to intervention that weaves systemic thinking and its post-modern influences with the cognitive and behavioural family intervention approaches. They position the user and family at the heart of the work, and attempt to develop a collaborative approach that assists the family members in negotiating the form and content of the meetings on a session by session basis. Their methods are based on the identification and interruption of unhelpful "interactional cycles" of behaviour and beliefs that may be seen to maintain problems, predicated on notions of circular causality. They hope to reduce experiences of blame, shame, and guilt by helping family members develop new perspectives in the context of a positive therapeutic alliance.

Chamberlain and Rosicky (1995) reviewed the family intervention studies for adolescents with severe conduct and delinquent problems and found that the family-based approaches reduced the problems compared with individual treatment approaches and no treatment. It is of interest that when families "dropped out" of treatment, or the intervention appeared to have no appreciable effect, there was a high correlation with family poverty and/or social isolation (high risk). Nugent *et al.*, (1993), in the Florida Network Study, showed that families designated as high risk were four times as likely to stay together after a family-based intervention than those who did not experience this, and those families who participated in more than five treatment sessions were twice as likely to stay together as families who had fewer sessions. So, for these high-risk families, family therapy may be a necessary component of the treatment package but is not sufficient in itself. All of this confirms the need for careful and sensitive convening and engagement of family members. Szapocnick and Williams (2000) have written about the difficulties in forming good working relationships with parents of children who have complex social, psychological and educational needs. Such research, while helpful in identifying the complexity of convening, could add to a sense of pessimism that the problems cannot be resolved.

In the UK, families designated as high risk are likely to be working with the three statutory agencies and, in addition may well be involved with the legal system. The child care professionals will need to coordinate their efforts with each other and to make working relationships with the family members. Campbell (1997) found that families working with a family therapy team as part of a child protection approach experienced strong fears that their children would be removed from their care. These fears made it difficult for both parents and professionals to develop trusting therapeutic relationships.

Van Roosmalen (2001) explored the development of the therapeutic alliance with a handful of families who could be described as having complex social, economic, and psychological needs, in a Tier Three intervention service. Using qualitative methods of interviewing and analysis, he identified some common themes to the experiences of parents and children. For example, the alliance was strengthened by an approach that took into account the developmental needs of the children and was child-centred in its approach; the alliance with the parents was strengthened by helping them shift their understandings of the causes of their family problems from a focus on the child to a more systemic understanding of causation; and the alliance was strengthened by the family members' perception of the therapist as genuinely interested in their points of view and experiences, thus enhancing their sense of participation in the work.

Multi-systemic therapy

Multi-systemic therapy (MST) was developed by Henggeler and colleagues (1998) in response to the need to work collaboratively and in partnership with families when adolescents present services and families with the challenge of serious clinical and legal problems. It is based on a social–ecological view that sees extra-familial systems as mutually interconnected to individuals and family groups in such a way that behaviour is seen as multi-determined. This ecological view is complementary to causal modelling studies of youth delinquency and substance abuse (Henggeler, 1997). For example, a combination of antisocial attitudes, low social support, harsh and inconsistent family discipline combined with low levels of child supervision, associating with similarly troubled and troublesome peers, lack of engagement with education and problems in school, and living in a neighbourhood with high levels of crime, are correlated highly with serious antisocial behaviour in adolescents.

MST is a family- and community-based approach that has demonstrated clinical utility as a cost-effective alternative to out-of-home placements for adolescents, such as in secure units or psychiatric units. The success of the approach is ascribed to a number of factors, which differentiate it from more common mental health and youth-offending team approaches. They include:

(a) providing services in family homes and other community settings;
(b) a package of interventions that comprehensively address the contextual and other determinants of the problems;
(c) a service philosophy that promotes collaboration with family members and is committed to working in partnership.

In particular, MST adheres to the following treatment principles:

(a) assessment that seeks to examine the fit between clinical problems and their wider systemic context;
(b) an emphasis on identifying systemic strengths in the group and encouraging what works well;
(c) interventions that are aimed at encouraging responsible behaviours and reducing irresponsible behaviours;
(d) interventions that are action oriented, in the here and now, and targeted to specifically defined problems;
(e) interventions that are targeted at behaviours between and within human systems that maintain the problem behaviours;
(f) interventions that are tailored to be developmentally appropriate;
(g) interventions that require family members to carry out "homework" tasks between meetings;
(h) evaluation of the effectiveness of the interventions from multiple vantage points, with the clinicians assuming the responsibility for overcoming obstacles to success;
(i) promotion of treatment maintenance and generalization by helping providers and carers address family members' needs across multiple systemic contexts.

The workload for a clinician who adheres to these multi-systemic principles is heavy. Nelson and Landsman (1992) recommend no more than five families per caseload, with a time-limited approach of 4—6 months, when working this way. The implications of this approach for training are enormous. At the very least, there is a requirement to obtain follow-up information about the outcomes of complex cases, with continuous quality assurance procedures.

We finish this discussion with a brief description of multi-family groups, which have a long tradition in systemic practice (Asen, 2002). These groups try to promote family members' own communicative abilities and competencies by creating an emotionally safe place within which the family groups can support each other. The rise of multi-family groups within the UK NHS suggests that systemic practice is finding its way into the treatment of some major "psychiatric" difficulties, such as eating disorders (Dare & Eisler, 2000) and major mental illness (Bishop *et al.*, 2002).

Historically, the multi-family group model was offered as a concurrent treatment, but has evolved as a sole therapy in its own right. Families act as consultants to other families, helping each other through sharing experiences, supporting coping, introducing new ideas, facilitating new styles of interaction, and so on. Two therapists, one more active, and one in a more reflective role, are often involved. Descriptions of the work suggest that families often do the work themselves, with therapists intervening if unhelpful dynamics develop, such as conflict between some parents. If this happens, other group members can be invited to reflect on the process, offering solutions, and a wider frame for understanding. Current developments incorporate reflecting processes and the notion of outsider witness groups (White, 1997).

Reflexive note

1. Consider your current practice as an individual therapist—what could you do differently in your work with individuals? How does thinking about, and working directly with, people's relationships help you think differently about your individual practice?

CHAPTER SEVEN

Integrative practice: thinking in the future

In this chapter we try to draw together the recursive themes of formulation, intervention, and evaluation. As we say at the outset, these three themes can be seen as an interlocking triangle in which each point of the triangle informs the other. Systemic thinking provides us with the framework within which we integrate diverse ideas. For us, the recursive loops between thinking and practice are grounded in pragmatic considerations of best fit and theory has never been about a search for a once-and-for-all understanding. Rather, it is more how we best describe and explain the circumstances under consideration, in terms of what we think we know, ever alert to new and disconfirmatory information. Our chief criterion for the evaluation of theory used for formulation is usefulness: how does this formulation best explain what is happening? from whose perspective? does it help us think further? does it guide our practice?

We have tried to present systemic formulation as a case study approach to practice-based evidence. We have argued that formulation offers a case by case approach to making theory evident in our clinical practice. For example, how our clinical observations are developed and evolve into progressive hypotheses that recursively inform our practice from the ground up, so to speak, much as in a grounded theory approach to practice, is made known through the practice of formulation. Formulation as a process thus enables evaluation, which itself is rooted in actual day to day practices. The collaborative approaches promoted within these pages parallel recent Department of Health research directives concerning user involvement in evaluation research. Arguably, a systemic approach helps us move beyond paying lip service to collaboration if formulation itself can be shown to be collaborative in nature.

The rapprochement with social constructionist critiques outlined here recognizes that formulation is not a static, one-size-fits-all process. The fit between understanding and practice is systemic at its heart. Feedback from clients and clinical experience informs thinking in a recursive loop with practice. This resembles a completed audit cycle in which a summary of the findings are presented back to service providers and users, changes are made to service delivery, feedback is elicited and presented back, and so on into another cycle. However, the recent turn to narrative among some systemic practitioners might be seen to challenge the necessity for, and the validity of formulation. For us, the process of formulation offers a way forward to narrative therapists interested in evaluation, through its grounding in practice-based-evidence.

We could not conclude this book without taking collaborative practice to task. We often ask whether we can actually be collaborative in our clinical practice, and if so, how. If we can argue that formulation is the vehicle for integrative practice, and the friend of evaluation, with collaborative practice valued and promoted as central to these triangular relationships, where might that take us? Many systemic practitioners are interested in reflective practices. These currently take many forms, ranging from the use of reflecting teams and in-room consultation practices to internal supervisory conversations. Team reflections can be viewed and reviewed with families after therapeutic sessions. We would suggest that these reflecting practices can be part of the process of formulation. For example, if we think of team reflections as early formulations, discussed in front of the family and with the family, thus including their views and feedback on the reflections, we begin to see how collaborative practice can evolve into dialectical formulation with families.

Specifically, we suggest that some of the following points follow from the approach that we have advocated, for example regarding the widespread use of reflecting teams in family therapy.

- It is helpful to keep in mind that our discussions are organized by the formulations of each member of the team.
- It is important to make explicit the assumptions underlying these discussions.
- Team members may assist each other in this process.
- We should try to keep what we say propositional rather than instructive.
- Our formulations should be on-going and formative.
- Each member of the team should try to maintain a critical and reflective position—to engage with our "internal supervisor".
- We should encourage a dialectical and collaborative conversation with our families.
- Creative ways of maintaining this collaborative stance should be sought: we might experiment with viewing and discussing video recordings of our reflecting discussions with families.

Many of these points are similar to those made by the Milan team regarding the value of "progressive hypothesizing". In effect we are saying that just as it is impossible for us not to communicate so, arguably, it is impossible for us not to formulate. Collaborative and ethical practice does not require that we abandon the need to engage in formulation, but that it is centre-stage in our thinking and practice. The alternative risks the danger of our work being based on intuition, prejudice, and mystification.

In conclusion, we wish to restate our commitment to, and passionate engagement with, systemic ideas. The revolution inherent in systemic thinking and practice, in which relational connections and context are held paramount, continue to inform our personal and professional lives.

REFERENCES

Alexander, J. F., Barton, C., Schiavo, R. S., & Parsons, B. V. (1976). Systems-behavioral intervention with families of delinquents: Therapist characteristics, family behavior, and outcome. *Journal of Consulting and Clinical Psychology, 44*: 656–664.

Amias, D. (2001). Personal communication.

Anderson, H., Goolishian, H. A., & Winderman, I. (1986). Problem determined systems. Toward transformation in family therapy. *Journal of Strategic and Family Therapy*, 4: 1–13.

Andersen, T. (1987). The reflecting team. Dialogue and meta-dialogue in clinical work. *Family Process, 26*: 415–428.

Aries, P. (1962). *Centuries of Childhood: A Social History of Family Life.* New York: Baldick.

Asen, E. (2002). Multiple family therapy: An overview. *Journal of Family Therapy, 24*(1): 3–16.

Bandura, M. M., & Goldman, C. (1995). Expanding the contextual analysis of clinical problems. *Cognitive and Behavioral Practice,* 2: 119–141.

Barkham, M. (1989). Exploratory therapy in 2+1 sessions: I. Rationale for a brief psychotherapy model. *British Journal of Psychotherapy,* 6: 81–88.

Bateson, G. (1972). *Steps to an Ecology of Mind.* New York: E. P. Dutton.

Bateson, G. (1980). *Mind and Nature: A Necessary Unity*. London: Fontana/Collins.

Bateson, G., Jackson, D. D., Haley, J., & Weakland, J. H. (1956). Towards a theory of schizophrenia. *Behavioural Science, 1*(4): 251–264.

Beavers, J., Hampson, R. B., Hulgus, Y. F., & Beavers, W. R. (1986). Coping in families with a retarded child. *Family Process, 25*: 365–378.

Beck, A. T. (1967). *Depression: Clinical, Experiential and Theoretical Aspects*. New York: Harper Row.

Bennun, I. (1989). Perceptions of the therapist in family therapy. *Journal of Family Therapy, 11*: 243–255.

Beresford, B. (1994). Resources and strategies: How parents cope with the care of a disabled child. *Journal of Child Psychology and Psychiatry, 35*: 171–209.

Berger, P. L., & Luckman, T. (1973). *The Social Construction of Reality*. Harmondsworth: Penguin.

Bergin, A. E., & Garfield, S. L. (Eds.) (1994). *Handbook of Psychotherapy and Behaviour Change: An Empirical Analysis* (4th edn). New York: Wiley.

Bishop, P., Clilverd, A., Cooklin, A., & Hunt, U. (2002). Mental health matters: A multi-family framework for mental health intervention. *Journal of Family Therapy, 24*(1): 31–45.

Black, D. (1987). Handicap and family therapy. In: A. Bentovim, G. Gorell Barnes & A. Cooklin (Eds.), *Family Therapy: Complementary Frameworks of Theory and Practice* (2nd edn). London: Academic Press.

Boscolo, L., & Bertrando, M. (1996). *Systemic Therapy with Individuals*. London: Karnac.

Boszormenyi-Nagy, I. (1987). *Foundations of Contextual Therapy: Collected Papers of Ivan Boszormenyi-Nagy*. New York: Brunner-Mazel.

Boyle, M. (1990). *Schizophrenia: A Scientific Delusion?* London: Routledge.

British Crime Survey (1996). *Home Office Statistical Bulletin*, Issue 19/96. Croydon: Home Office.

British Crime Survey (2000). *Home Office Statistical Bulletin*, Issue 18/00. Croydon: Home Office.

Brody, G. (Ed.) (1996). *Sibling Relationships: Their Causes and Consequences*. Jersey City, New Jersey: Ablex.

Browne, K., & Herbert, M. (1997). *Preventing Family Violence*. Chichester: Wiley.

Bruch, H. (1978). *The Golden Cage*. Cambridge, MA: Harvard University Press.

Bruner, J. (1990). *Acts of Meaning*. London: Harvard University Press.

Brunning, H., & Huffington, C. (1990). Jumping off the fence: Developing the consultancy model. *Clinical Psychology Forum, 29*: 31–33.

Bryant-Waugh, R., & Lask, B. (1995). Eating disorders—an overview. *Journal of Family Therapy, 17*: 13–30.

Burbach, F. R., & Stanbridge, R. I. (1998). A family intervention in psychosis service integrating the systemic and family management approaches. *Journal of Family Therapy, 20*(3): 311–325.

Burck, C., & Speed, B. (Eds.) (1995). *Gender, Power and Relationships*. London: Routledge.

Burck, C., Frosh, S., Strickland-Clark, L., & Morgan, K. (1998). The process of enabling change: A study of therapist interventions in family therapy. *Journal of Family Therapy, 20*(3): 253–267.

Burnham, J. B. (1986). *Family Therapy. First Steps Towards a Systemic Approach*. London: Tavistock.

Byng-Hall, J. (1995). *Rewriting Family Scripts: Improvisation and Systems Change*. New York: Guilford Press.

Byng-Hall, J. (1998). Evolving ideas about narrative: Re-editing the re-editing of family mythology. *Journal of Family Therapy, 20*(2): 133–143.

Byng-Hall, J. (2000). Therapist reflections. Diverse developmental pathways for the family. *Journal of Family Therapy, 22*: 264–272.

Byrne, E., Cunningham, C., & Sloper, P. (1988). *Families and their Children with Down's Syndrome: One Feature in Common*. London: Routledge.

Campbell, D. (1995). *Learning Consultation: A Systemic Framework*. London: Karnac.

Campbell, D. (1997). The other side of the story: The client's experience of therapy. In: R. Papadopoulos & J. Byng-Hall (Eds.), *Multiple Voices: Narrative in Systemic Family Psychotherapy*. London: Gerald Duckworth & Co.

Campbell, D. (1999). Family therapy and beyond: Where is the Milan systemic approach today? *Child Psychology and Psychiatry Review, 4*: 76–84.

Campbell, D. (2001). *The Social Construction of Organizations*. London: Karnac.

Campbell, D., Draper, R., & Huffington, C. (1991). *A Systemic Approach to Consultation*. London: Karnac Books.

Carpenter, J., & Treacher, A. (1989). *Problems and Solutions in Marital and Family Therapy*. Oxford: Blackwell.

Carr, A. (1997). *Family Therapy and Systemic Consultation*. Lanham, MD: University Press of America.

Carr, A. (1999). *The Handbook of Child and Adolescent Clinical Psychology: A Contextual Approach*. London: Routledge.

Carr, A. (2000a). Evidence-based practice in family therapy and systemic consultation I. *Journal of Family Therapy, 22*(1): 29–60.

Carr, A. (2000b). Evidence-based practice in family therapy and systemic consultation II. *Journal of Family Therapy, 22*(3): 273–295.

Carter, E., & McGoldrick, M. (1989). *The Changing Family Life Cycle* (2nd edn). Boston, MA: Allyn & Bacon.

Cecchin, G. (1987). Hypothesizing, circularity and neutrality revisited: an invitation to curiosity. *Family Process, 26*(4): 405–414.

Cederborg, A. (1997). Young children's participation in family therapy talk. *The American Journal of Family Therapy, 25*: 28–38.

Chamberlain, P., & Rosicky, J. G. (1995). The effectiveness of family therapy in the treatment of adolescents with conduct disorders and delinquency. *Journal of Marital and Family Therapy, 21*: 441–459.

Cottrell, D., & Boston, P., (2002). The effectiveness of systemic family therapy for children and adolescents. *Journal of Child Psychology and Psychiatry, 43*: 573–586.

Coulahan, M. (1995). Being a therapist in eating disorder treatment trials: constraints and creativity. *Journal of Family Therapy, 17*(1): 79–96.

Dale, N. (1996). *Working with Families of Children with Special Needs: Partnership and Practice*. London: Routledge.

Dallos, R. (1991). *Family Belief Systems, Therapy and Change*. Buckingham: Open University Press.

Dallos, R. (1997). *Interacting Stories, Narratives, Family Beliefs and Therapy*. London: Karnac.

Dallos, R. (2001). ANT—Attachment Narrative Therapy: Narrative and attachment theory approaches in systemic family therapy. *Journal of Family Psychotherapy, 12*: 43–72.

Dallos, S., & Dallos, R. (1997). *Couples, Sex and Power: The Politics of Desire*. Buckingham: Open University Press.

Dallos, R., & Draper, R. (2000). *An Introduction to Family Therapy: Systemic Theory and Practice*. Milton Keynes: Open University Press.

Dallos, R., & Hamilton-Brown, L. (2000). Pathways to problems—an exploratory study of how problems evolve vs dissolve in families. *Journal of Family Therapy, 22*: 375–393.

Dallos, R., & Urry, A. (1999). Abandoning our parents and grandparents: Does social construction mean the end of systemic family therapy? *Journal of Family Therapy, 21*: 161–186.

D'Ardenne, P., & Mahtani, A. (1999). *Transcultural Counselling in Action* (2nd edn). London: Sage.

Dare, C., & Eisler, I. (2000). A multi-family group day treatment programme for adolescent eating disorder. *European Eating Disorders Review, 8*: 4–18.

Department of Health (1996). *Clinical Guidelines: Using Clinical Guidelines to Improve Patient Care within the NHS.* Leeds: NGS Executive.

Dimmock, B., & Dungworth, D. (1985). Beyond the family: Using network meetings with statutory child care cases. *Journal of Family Therapy, 7*: 45–68.

Dobash, R. E., & Dobash, R. P. (1992). *Women, Violence and Social Change.* London: Routledge.

Domestic Abuse Intervention Project (1987). *Year End Report to Department of Corrections, 1987.* Duluth, MN: Author (DAIP, 206 W. 4th Street, Duluth, MN 55806, USA).

Dowling, E. (1979). Co-therapy: A clinical researcher's view. In: S. Walrond-Skinner (Ed.), *Family and Marital Psychotherapy: A Critical Approach* (pp. 173–199). London: Routledge and Kegan Paul.

Dowling, E., & Osborne, E. (1994). *The Family and the School: A Joint Systems Approach to Problems with Children* (2nd edn). London: Routledge.

Duncan, B., & Miller, S. (2000). *The Heroic Client: Doing client-directed, outcome informed therapy.* San Francisco: Jossey-Bass.

Dunst, C. J., Trivette, C. M., & Deal, A. G. (1994). *Supporting and Strengthening Families, Vol. I. Methods, Strategies and Practices.* Cambridge, MA: Brookline Books.

Duvall, E. (1957). *Family Development.* Philadelphia: Lippincott.

Edwards, M., & Steinglass, P. (1995). Family therapy treatment outcomes for alcoholism. *Journal of Marital and Family Therapy, 21*: 475–509.

Ehrensaft, M., & Vivian, D. (1996). Spouses' reasons for not reporting existing marital aggression as a marital problem. *Journal of Family Psychology, 10*: 443–453.

Elliott, R. (1984). A discovery-oriented approach to significant events in psychotherapy: Interpersonal process recall and comprehensive process analysis. In: L. Rice & L. Greenbergs (Eds.), *Patterns of Change* (pp. 49–72). New York: Guilford Press.

Elliott, R., & Shapiro, D. A. (1992). Clients and therapists as analysts of significant events. In: S. G. Tonkmanian & D. L. Rennie (Eds.), *Psychotherapy Process Research, Paradigmatic Narrative Approaches* (pp. 163–186). Newbury Park, CA: Sage.

Emmelkamp, P., & Foa, E. (1983). Failures are a challenge. In: E. Foa & P. Emmelkamp (Eds.), *Failures in Behavior Therapy*. New York: Wiley.

Epstein, N., Bishop, D., Ryan, C., Miller, I., & Keitner, J. (1993). The McMaster Model: View of healthy family functioning. In: F. Walsh (Ed.), *Normal Family Processes* (2nd edn). New York: Guilford Press.

Erickson, E. (1968). *Identity, Youth and Crisis*. New York: Norton.

Eron, J. B., & Lund, T. W. (1993). How problems evolve and dissolve. Integrating narrative and strategic concepts. *Family Process, 32*: 291–309.

Fadden, G. (1998). Research update: psychoeducational family interventions. *Journal of Family Therapy, 20*(3): 293–309.

Fairburn, G., & Brownell, I. (2002). *Eating Disorders and Obesity* (2nd edn). New York: Guilford Press.

Feeney, J., & Noller, P. (1996). *Adult Attachment*. London: Sage.

Fernando, S. (1991). *Mental Health, Race and Culture*. London: Macmillan Mind Publications.

Fiddell, B. (2000). Exploring the use of family therapy with adults with a learning disability. *Journal of Family Therapy, 22*(3): 308–323.

Fishman, P. (1983). Interaction, the work women do. In: B. Thorne, C. Kramarae & N. Henley (Eds.), *Language, Gender and Society*. Rowley, MA: Newbury House.

Folkman, S., & Lazarus, R. (1980). An analysis of coping in a middle-aged community sample. *Journal of Health and Social Behavior, 21*: 219–239.

Foucault, M. (1975). *The Archeology of Knowledge*. London: Tavistock.

Foucault, M. (1980). *Power/Knowledge: Selected Interviews and Other Writings*. New York: Harvester Wheatsheaf.

Fox, D., & Prilleltensky, I. (Eds.) (1997). *Critical Psychology: An Introduction*. London: Sage.

Fraser, S. (1995). Process, problems, and solutions in brief therapy. *Journal of Marital and Family Therapy, 21*(3): 265–279.

Fredman, G. (1997). *Death Talk: Conversations with Children and Families*. London: Karnac.

Friedlander, M. L., Wildman, J., Heatherington, L., & Skowron, E. A.

(1994). What we do and don't know about the process of family therapy. *Journal of Family Psychology, 8*: 390–416.

Frosh, S. (1997). Postmodern narratives: Or muddles in the mind. In: R. Papadopoulos & J. Byng-Hall (Eds.), *Multiple Voices: Narrative in Systemic Family Psychotherapy*. London: Gerald Duckworth & Co.

Frosh, S., Burck, C., Strickland-Clark, L., & Morgan, K. (1996). Engaging with change: A process study of family therapy. *Journal of Family Therapy, 18*: 141–161.

Frude, N. (1991). *Understanding Family Problems: A Psychological Approach*. Chichester: John Wiley & Sons.

Gath, A., & Gumley, D. (1987). Retarded children and their siblings. *Journal of Child Psychology and Psychiatry, 28*: 715–730.

Geffner, R., & Pagelow, M. (1999) Victims of spouse abuse. In: R. Ammerman & M. Hersen (Eds.), *Assessment of Family Violence: A Clinical and Legal Sourcebook* (2nd edn) (pp. 113–135) . New York: Wiley.

Gelles, R., & Cornell, C. (1990). *Intimate Violence in Families*. Newbury Park, CA: Sage.

Gergen, K. J. (1982). *Toward Transformation in Social Knowledge*. New York: Springer.

Gergen, K. J. (1985). The social constructionist movement in modern psychology. *American Psychologist, 40*: 266–275.

Gilligan, C. (1982). *In a Different Voice*. Cambridge: Harvard University Press.

Goffman, E. (1971). *Asylums*. Harmondsworth: Penguin.

Goldberg, D., Magrill, L., Hale, J., Damaskinidou, K., Paul, J., & Tham, S. (1995). Protection and loss: working with learning disabled adults and their families. *Journal of Family Therapy, 17*: 263–280.

Goldner, V., Penn, P., Sheinberg, M., & Walker, G. (1990). Love and violence: paradoxes of volatile attachments. *Family Process, 29*: 343–364.

Goldstein, M., & Miklowitz, D. (1995). The effectiveness of psychoeducational family therapy in the treatment of schizophrenic disorders. *Journal of Marital and Family Therapy, 21*: 361–376.

Goodyer, I. (1990). *Life Experiences, Development, and Childhood Psychopathology*. Chichester: Wiley.

Gorell Barnes, J., Thompson, P., Daniel, G., & Burchardt, N. (1998). *Growing Up in Step-families*. Oxford: Clarendon Press.

Greenberg, L. S. (1986). Change process research. *Journal of Consulting and Clinical Psychology, 54*: 4–9.

Gregory, M., & Leslie, L. (1996). Different lenses: Variations in clients' perception of family therapy by race and gender. *Journal of Marital and Family Therapy, 22*: 239–251.

Gurman, A. S., & Kniskern, D. P. (1978). Research on marital and family therapy: progress, perspectives and prospects. In: S. L. Garfield & A. E. Bergin (Eds.), *Handbook of Psychotherapy and Behaviour Change: An Empirical Analysis* (2nd edn) (pp. 817–902). New York: Wiley.

Gurman, A. S., Kniskern, D. P., & Pinsof, W. (1986). Research on the process and outcome of marital and family therapy. In: S. L. Garfield & A. E. Bergin (Eds.), *Handbook of Psychotherapy and Behavior Change* (3rd edn) (pp. 565–624). New York: Wiley.

Halevy, J. (1998). A genogram with an attitude. *Journal of Marital and Family Therapy, 24*(2): 233–242.

Haley, J. (1969). *The Power Tactics of Jesus Christ and Other Essays*. New York: Grossman.

Haley, J. (1973). *Uncommon Therapy: Psychiatric Techniques of Milton H. Erickson, M.D.* New York: Norton.

Haley, J. (1976). *Problem-solving Therapy*. San Francisco: Jossey Bass.

Hampson, R., & Beavers, R. (1996). Family therapy and outcome: Relationships between therapist and family styles. *Contemporary Family Therapy, 18*: 345–370.

Hardwick, P. (1991). Families and the professional network: An attempted classification of professional network actions which can hinder change. *Journal of Family Therapy, 13*: 187–206.

Hardy, K. V., & Laszloffy, T. A. (1995). The cultural genogram: Key to training culturally competent family therapists. *Journal of Marital and Family Therapy, 21*: 227–237.

Hare Mustin, R. (1986). The problem of gender in family therapy theory. *Family Process, 26*: 15–27.

Harre, R., & Secord, P. (1972). *The Explanation of Social Behaviour*. Oxford: Blackwell.

Hatton, C., Hastings, R., & Vetere, A. (1999). Psychology and people with learning disabilities: A case for inclusion? *The Psychologist, 12*: 231–232.

Hayward, M. (1996). Is second order practice possible? *Journal of Family Therapy, 18*: 219–242.

Hazelrigg, M. D., Cooper, H. M., & Borduin, C. M. (1987). Evaluating the effectiveness of family therapies: An integrative review and analysis. *Psychological Bulletin, 101*: 428–442.

Hearn, J. (1994). Making sense of men and men's violence to women. *Clinical Psychology Forum, 64*: 13–16.

Henggeler, S. (1997). The development of effective drug abuse services for youth. In: J. Egerertson, D. Fox & A. Leshner (Eds.), *Treating Drug Abusers Effectively* . New York: Blackwell.

Henggeler, S., Schoenwald, S., Borduin, C., Rowland, M., & Cunningham, P. (1998). *Multisystemic Treatment of Antisocial Behaviour in Children and Adolescents.* New York: Guilford Press.

Hoffman, L. (1993). *Exchanging Voices: A Collaborative Approach to Family Therapy.* London: Karnac.

Hoffman, L. (1998). A constructivist position for family therapy. *The Irish Journal of Psychology, 9*: 110–129.

Hoffman, L., & Long, L. (1969). A systems dilemma. *Family Process, 8*: 211–234.

Hollway, W. (1989). *Subjectivity and Method in Psychology.* London: Sage.

Holtzworth-Munroe, A., & Hutchinson, G. (1993). Attributing negative intent to wife behavior: The attributions of partially violent versus non-violent men. *Journal of Abnormal Psychology, 102*: 206–211.

Homans, G. (1961). *Social Behaviour: Its Elementary Forms.* New York: Harcourt Brace Jovanovich.

Howe, D. (1989). *The Consumer's View of Family Therapy.* London: Gower.

Jackson, D. (1957). The question of family homeostasis. *Psychiatry Quarterly Supplement, 31*: 79–99.

James, K. (1996). Truth or fiction: Men as victims of domestic violence? *Australia and New Zealand Journal of Family Therapy, 17*: 121–125.

Jenkins, A. (1990). *Invitations to Responsibility.* Adelaide, SA: Dulwich Centre Publications.

Jenkins, H., & Asen, E. (1992). Family therapy without the family: A framework for systemic practice. *Journal of Family Therapy, 9*: 3–25.

Johnson, M. (1995). Patriarchal terrorism and common couple violence: two forms of violence against women. *Journal of Marriage and the Family, 57*: 283–294.

Johnstone, L. (1993). Are we allowed to disagree? *Clinical Psychology Forum, 56*: 31–34.

Jones, E. (1991). *Working With Adult Survivors of Child Sexual Abuse.* London: Karnac.

Jones, E., & Asen, E. (2000). *Systemic Couple Therapy and Depression.* London: Karnac.

Jory, B., & Anderson, D. (2000). Intimate justice III: Healing the anguish of abuse and embracing the anguish of accountability. *Journal of Marital and Family Therapy, 26*(3): 329–340.

Kant, I. (1791). *Critique of Pure Reason*. Basingstoke, Hants: MacMillan Press.

Kelly, G. A. (1955). *The Psychology of Personal Constructs, Vols. I & II*. New York: Norton.

Kent, R. (1990). Focusing on women. In: S. Collins (Ed.), *Alcohol, Social Work, and Helping*. London: Routledge.

Kerr, M. E., & Bowen, M. (1988). *Family Evaluation: An Approach Based on Bowen Theory*. New York: Norton.

Kingston, P., & Smith, D. (1983). Preparation for live consultation and live supervision when working without a one-way screen. *Journal of Family Therapy, 5*: 219–233.

Korzybski, A. (1942). *Science and Sanity: An Introduction to Non-Aristotelian Systems and General Semantics*. Lancaster, PA: Science Books.

Kuehl, B. P., Newfield, N. A., & Joanning, H. (1990). A client-based description of family therapy. *Journal of Family Psychology, 3*: 310–321.

Lamb, M., & Billings, L. (1997). Fathers with children with special needs. In: M. Lamb (Ed.), *The Role of the Father in Child Development* (3rd edn) (pp. 179–190). New York: Wiley.

Larner, G. (2000). Towards a common ground in psychoanalysis and family therapy. On knowing not to know. *Journal of Family Therapy, 22*(1): 61–82.

Le Grange, D., Eisler, I., Dare, C., & Russell, G. (1992). Evaluation of family treatments in adolescent anorexia nervosa: A pilot study. *International Journal of Eating Disorders, 12*: 347–357.

Leff, J., Vearnals, S., Brewin, C., Wolff, G., Alexander, B., Asen, E., Dayson, D., Jones, E., Chisholm, D., & Everitt, B. (2000). The London Depression Intervention Trial: An RCT of antidepressants versus couple therapy in the treatment and maintenance of depressed people with a partner: Clinical outcomes and costs. *British Journal of Psychiatry, 177*: 95–100.

Lieberman, S. (1979). *Transgenerational Family Therapy*. London: Croom Helm.

Llewelyn, S. (1988). Psychological therapy as viewed by clients and therapists. *British Journal of Clinical Psychology, 27*: 105–114.

Lynggaard, H., Dontai, S., Pearce, P., & Sklavounos, D. (2001). A difference that made a difference: Introducing systemic ideas and practices into a multi-disciplinary learning disability service. *Clinical Psychology*, *3*: 12–15.

Manojlovic, J., & Partridge, K. (2001). A framework for systemic consultation with acute ward systems. *Clinical Psychology*, *3*: 27–30.

Markus, E., Lange, A., & Pettigrew, T. (1990). Effectiveness of family therapy: A meta-analysis. *Journal of Family Therapy*, *12*: 205–221.

Martin, S. (1989). *The Child Development Centre: A Consumer Perspective*. Report commissioned by The Spastics Society in support of the establishment of Child Development Centres.

Marx, K. (1967). *The Communist Manifesto*. New York: Lasky.

Mas, C., Alexander, J., & Barton, C. (1985). Modes of expression in family therapy: A process study of roles and gender. *Journal of Marital and Family Therapy*, *11*: 411–415.

McGoldrick, M., & Gerson, R. (1989). Genograms and the family life-cycle. In: B. Carter & M. McGoldrick (Eds.), *The Changing Family Life Cycle* (2nd edn) (pp. 164–189). Boston: Allyn and Bacon.

McGoldrick, M., Preto, N., Hines, P., & Lee, E. (1991). Ethnicity and family therapy. In: A. S. Gurman & D. P. Kniskern (Eds.), *Handbook of Family Therapy, Vol. II*. New York: Brunner Mazel.

McHale, E., & Carr, A. (1998). The effect of supervisor and trainee therapist gender on supervision discourse. *Journal of Family Therapy*, *20*: 395–411.

Mead, G. H. (1934). *Mind, Self and Society*. Chicago: University of Chicago Press.

Miller, S., & Berg, I. (1995). *The Miracle Method: A Radically New Approach to Problem Drinking*. New York: Norton.

Miller, W., & Rollnick, S. (1991). *Motivational Interviewing: Preparing People to Change Addictive Behaviour*. New York: Guilford Press.

Minuchin, S. (1974). *Families and Family Therapy*. Cambridge, MA: Harvard University Press.

Minuchin, S., Rosman, B., & Baker, L. (1978). *Psychosomatic Families: Anorexia Nervosa in Context*. Cambridge, MA: Harvard University Press.

Minuchin, S., Lee, W-Y., & Simon, M. (1996). *Mastering Family Therapy: Journeys of Growth and Transformation*. Chichester: Wiley.

Moffitt, T., & Caspi, A. (1998). Annotation: Implications of violence between intimate partners for child psychologists and psychiatrists. *Journal of Child Psychology and Psychiatry*, *39*: 137–144.

Motz, A. (2001). *The Psychology of Female Violence: Crimes Against the Body*. Hove: Brunner-Routledge.

Nelson, K. E., & Landsman, M. J. (1992). *Alternative Models of Family Preservation: Family-based Services in Context*. Springfield, IL: Charles Thomas.

Nelson-Jones, R. (1988). *Practical Counselling and Helping Skills*. London: Cassell.

Nock, S. L. (2000). The divorce of marriage and parenthood. *Journal of Family Therapy, 22*: 245–263.

Novaco, R. (1975). *Anger Control: The Development and Evaluation of an Experimental Treatment*. Lexington, MA: Lexington Books.

NSPCC (1985). Child abuse deaths. *Information Briefing No. 5*. London: NSPCC.

Nugent, W. R., Carpenter, D., & Parks, J. (1993). A statewide evaluation of family preservation and family reunification services. *Research on Social Work Practice, 3*: 40–65.

O'Brien, M. (1990). The place of men in a gender-sensitive therapy. In: R. J. Perelberg & A. C. Miller (Eds.), *Gender and Power in Families* (pp. 195–208). London: Routledge.

O'Hanlon, B. (1994). The third wave. *Family Therapy Networker, 18*: 18–29.

Olson, D. (2000). Circumplex model of marital and family interaction. *Journal of Family Therapy, 22*: 144–167.

Orford, J., & Harwin, J. (Eds.) (1982). *Alcohol and the Family*. London: Croom Helm.

Patterson, G. R., & Chamberlain, P. (1988). Treatment process: A problem at three levels. In: L. C. Wynne (Ed.), *The State of the Art in Family Therapy Research: Controversies and Recommendations* (pp. 189–226). New York: Family Process Press.

Patterson, G. R., & Forgatch, M. S. (1985). Therapist behavior as a determinant for client non-compliance: A paradox for the behavior modifier. *Journal of Consulting and Clinical Psychology, 53*: 846–851.

Penfold, P. S., & Walker, G. A. (1984). *Women and the Psychiatric Paradox*. Milton Keynes: Open University Press.

Penn, P. (1985). Feed-forward: Future questions, future maps. *Family Process, 24*: 299–310.

Perlesz, A., Furlong, M., & The "D" Family. (1996). A systemic therapy unravelled: In through the out door. In: C. Flaskas & A. Perlesz (Eds.), *The Therapeutic Relationship in Systemic Therapy*. London: Karnac.

Phoenix, A. (2001). *Racialisation of everyday life*. Lecture given to Masters in Systemic Psychotherapy. Tavistock Centre: London.

Pilgrim, D. (2000). The real problem for postmodernism. *Journal of Family Therapy, 22*: 6–23

Pinsof, W. M., & Catherall, D. R. (1986). The integrative psychotherapy alliance: Family, couple and individual therapy scales. *Journal of Marital and Family Therapy, 12*: 132–151.

Pinsof, W. M., & Wynne, L. (1995). The efficacy of marital and family therapy: An empirical overview, conclusions and recommendations. *Journal of Marital and Family Therapy, 21*: 585–613.

Pinsof, W. M., & Wynne, L. (2000). Toward progress research: Closing the gap between family therapy practice and research. *Journal of Marital and Family Therapy, 26*: 1–8.

Plomin, R. (1986). *Development, Genetics and Psychology*. Hillsdale, NJ: Lawrence Erlbaum.

Pocock, D. (1996). Comment: Reconciling the given and the made. *Journal of Family Therapy, 18*: 249–254.

Postner, R., Guttman, H., Sigal, J., Epstein, N., & Rakoff, V. (1971). Process and outcome in conjoint family therapy. *Family Process, 10*: 451–474.

Potter, J., & Wetherell, M. (1987). *Discourse and Social Psychology: Beyond Attitudes and Behaviour*. London: Sage.

Prochaska, J., & DiClemente, C. (1992). Stages of change in the modification of problem behaviors. In: M. Herson, R. M. Eisler & P. M. Miller (Eds.), *Progress in Behavior*. Sycamore, IL: Sycamore Press.

Procter, H. G. (1981). Family construct psychology. An approach to understanding and treating families. In: S. Walrond-Skinner (Ed.), *Developments in Family Therapy*. London: Routledge & Kegan Paul.

Procter, H. G. (1985). A construct approach to family therapy and systems intervention. In: E. Button (Ed.), *Personal Construct Theory and Mental Health*. Beckenham: Croom Helm.

Procter, H. G. (1996) The family construct system. In: D. Kalekin-Fishman & B. Walker (Eds.), *The Construction of Group Realities: Culture, Society and Personal Construct Psychology*. London: Krieger.

Quine, L., & Pahl, J. (1989). *Stress and Coping in Families Caring for a Child with Severe Mental Handicap: A Longitudinal Survey*. University of Kent at Canterbury: Institute of Social and Applied Psychology and Centre for Health Service Studies.

Radcliffe Richards, J. (1980). *The Sceptical Feminist*. Harmondsworth: Penguin.

Reder, P. (1986). Multi-agency family systems. *Journal of Family Therapy, 8*: 139–152.

Reder, P., & Lucey, C. (Eds.) (1995). *Assessment of Parenting: Psychiatric and Psychological Contributions*. London: Routledge.

Reder, P., & Fredman, G. (1996). The relationship to help: Interacting beliefs about the treatment process. *Clinical Child Psychology and Psychiatry, 1*: 457–467.

Reimers, S. (1999). "Good morning, Sir!" "Axe handle." Talking at cross-purposes in family therapy. *Journal of Family Therapy, 21*: 360–376.

Reimers, S. (2001). Understanding alliances: How can research inform user-friendly practice? *Journal of Family Therapy, 23*(1): 46–62.

Reimers, S., & Treacher, A. (1995). *Introducing User-friendly Family Therapy*. London: Routledge.

Reiss, D. (1980). *The Family's Construction of Reality*. London: Routledge & Kegan Paul.

Saunders, D. (1986). When battered women use violence: Husband abuse or self-defense. *Violence and Victims, 1*: 47–60.

Schaffer, H. R. (1977). *Studies in Infancy*. London: Academic Press.

Scharff, D., & Scharff, J. (1987). *Object Relations Family Therapy*. New York: Jason Aronson.

Selvini-Palazzoli, M. (1974). *Self-starvation*. London: Human Context Books.

Selvini-Palazzoli, M., Boscolo, L., Cecchin, G., & Prata, G. (1980a). The problem of the referring person. *Journal of Marital and Family Therapy, 6*: 3–9.

Selvini-Palazzoli, M., Boscolo, L., Cecchin, G., & Prata, G. (1980b). Hypothesizing–circularity–neutrality: Three guidelines for the conductor of the session. *Family Process, 19*(1): 3–12.

Selvini-Palazzoli, M., Cecchin, G., Prata, G., & Boscolo, L. (1978). *Paradox and Counter Paradox: A New Model in the Therapy of the Family in Schizophrenic Transaction*. New York: Jason Aronson.

Shadish, W. R., Ragsdale, K., Glaser, R. R., & Montgomery, L. M. (1995). The efficacy and effectiveness of marital and family therapy: A perspective from meta-analysis. *Journal of Marital and Family Therapy, 21*: 345–360.

Shalan, D., & Griggs, H. (1998). The age of consent: involving children in their own referral process. *Clinical Psychology Forum, 116*: 19–23.

Shapiro, R. J. (1974). Therapist attitudes and premature termination in family and individual therapy. *Journal of Nervous and Mental Disease, 159*: 101–107.

Shields, C. G., Sprenkle, D. H., & Constantine, J. A. (1991). Anatomy of an initial interview: The importance of joining and structuring skills. *American Journal of Family Therapy, 19*: 318.

Skynner, R. (1976). *One Flesh: Separate Persons: Principles of Family and Marital Psychotherapy*. London: Constable.

Slade, P. (1982). Towards a functional analysis of anorexia nervosa and bulimia nervosa. *British Journal of Clinical Psychology, 21*: 167–179.

Sloper, P. (1989). *Families and their children with Down's Syndrome*. Paper presented at the BIMH Conference, Keele.

Sloper, P. (1999). Models of service support for parents of disabled children. What do we know? What do we need to know? *Child: Care, Health and Development, 25*: 85–99.

Smale, J. (1978). *Shared care: Support services for families with handicapped children*. Paper read at Voluntary Council for Handicapped Children, Coventry.

Squire-Dehouck, B. (1993). Evaluation of conjoint family therapy versus family counselling in adolescent anorexic patients: a two-year follow-up study. Unpublished Dissertation, Diploma of Psychology, British Psychological Society, London.

Stainton-Rogers, R., & Stainton-Rogers, W. (1992). *Stories of Childhood*. New York: Harvester Wheatsheaf.

Stenfert-Kroese, B., Dagnan, D., & Lounidis, K. (Eds.) (1997). *Cognitive Behaviour Therapy for People with Learning Disabilities*. Routledge: London.

Stern, D. (1985). *The Interpersonal World of the Infant*. New York: Basic Books.

Stith, S. M., Rosen, K. H., McCollum, E. E., Coleman, J. U., & Herman, S. A. (1996). The voices of children: preadolescent children's experiences in family therapy. *Journal of Marital and Family Therapy, 22*: 69–86.

Stratford, J. (1998). Women and men in conversation: a consideration of therapists' interruptions in therapeutic discourse. *Journal of Family Therapy, 20*(4): 383–394.

Straus, M. A. (1994). *Violence in the Lives of Adolescents*. New York: Norton.

Straus, M. A., & Gelles, R. J. (1990). *Physical Violence in American Families: Risk Factors and Adaptations to Violence in 8,145 Families*. New Brunswick, NJ: Transaction Publishers.

Street, E., Downey, J., & Brazier, A. (1991). The development of therapeutic consultations in child-focused family work. *Journal of Family Therapy, 13*: 311–334.

Strickland-Clark, L., Campbell, D., & Dallos, D. (2000). Children's and adolescents' views on family therapy. *Journal of Family Therapy, 22*(3): 324–341.

Szapocnick, J., & Williams, R. A. (2000). Brief strategic family therapy: Twenty-five years of interplay among theory, research and practice in adolescent behavior problems and drug abuse. *Clinical Child and Family Psychology Review, 3*: 117–134.

Tew, B. (1974). Must a family with a handicapped child be a handicapped family? *Developmental Medicine and Child Neurology, 16*: 95–98.

Tomm, K. (1984a). One perspective on the Milan systemic approach: Part I. Overview of development, theory and practice. *Journal of Marital and Family Therapy, 10*(2): 113–125.

Tomm, K. (1984b). One perspective on the Milan systemic approach: Part II. Description of session format, interviewing style and interventions. *Journal of Marital and Family Therapy, 10*(3): 253–271.

Tomm, K., & Wright, L. (1979). Training in family therapy: Perceptual, conceptual and executive skills. *Family Process, 28*: 227–250.

Treacher, A., & Carpenter, J. (1983). On the failure to take convening strategies seriously—a reply to Campion. *Journal of Family Therapy, 5*: 259–262.

Trevarthen, C. (1980). The foundations of inter-subjectivity: development of interpersonal and co-operative understanding. In: D. Olson (Ed.), *Essays in Honour of J. S. Bruner*. New York: Norton.

Trute, B., & Hauch, C. (1988). Building on family strength: A study of families with positive adjustment to the birth of a developmentally disabled child. *Journal of Marital and Family Therapy, 14*: 185–193.

Turner, W. (2001). Cultural considerations in developing research programmes. *Journal of Primary Prevention, 21*: 285–303.

Van Roosmalen, M. (2001). Therapist intervention factors that influence therapeutic alliance events in family therapy with multi-problem families: a qualitative study. Unpublished Dissertation, Doctorate in Clinical Psychology, Canterbury Christ Church University College.

Vaughan, C., & Leff, J. (1976). The measurement of expressed emotion in the families of psychiatric patients. *British Journal of Social and Clinical Psychology, 15*: 157–165.

Velleman, R. (1992). "Oh, my drinking doesn't affect them": Families of problem drinkers. *Clinical Psychology Forum, 48*: 6–10.

Velleman, R., Copello, A., & Maslin, J. (Eds.) (1998). *Living with Drink: Women Who Live with Problem Drinkers*. London: Longman.

Vetere, A. (1993). Family therapy in services for people with learning difficulties. In: J. Carpenter & A. Treacher (Eds.), *Using Family Therapy in the 90s* (pp. 111–130). Oxford: Blackwell.

Vetere, A. (1996). The neglect of family systems ideas and practice in services for children and young people with learning disabilities. *Clinical Child Psychology and Psychiatry, 1*: 485–488.

Vetere, A. (1998). A family systems perspective. In: R. Velleman, A. Copello & J. Maslin (Eds.), *Living with Drink: Women Who Live with Problem Drinkers* (pp. 113–127). London: Longman.

Vetere, A., & Cooper, J. (2001). Working systemically with family violence: risk, responsibility and collaboration. *Journal of Family Therapy, 23*(4): 378–396.

Vetere, A., & Cooper, J. (2003). Setting up a domestic violence service. *Child and Adolescent Mental Health, 8*: 61–67.

Vetere, A., & Gale, A. (1987). *Ecological Studies of Family Life*. Chichester: Wiley.

Vetere, A., & Henley, M. (2001). Integrating couples and family therapy into a community alcohol service. A pantheoretical approach. *Journal of Family Therapy, 23*: 85–101.

Vetere, M., & Henley, M. (2002). The weave of object relations and family systems thinking: Working therapeutically with families and couples in a community alcohol service. In: I. Safvestad-Nolan & P. Nolan (Eds.), *Object Relations and Integrative Psychotherapy: Tradition and Innovation in Theory and Practice* (pp. 111–125). London: Whurr.

von Bertalanffy, L. (1968). *General System Theory: Foundation, Development, Application*. New York: Brazillier.

Wachtel, E. F., & Wachtel, P. L. (1986). *Family Dynamics in Individual Psychotherapy: A Guide to Clinical Strategies*. New York: Guilford Press.

Waldegrave, C. T. (1990). Just therapy. *Dulwich Centre Newsletter, 1*: 5–46.

Walrond-Skinner, S., & Watson, D. (1987). *Ethical Issues in Family Therapy*. London: Routledge and Kegan Paul.

Walters, J., Tasker, F., & Bichard, S. (2001). "Too busy?" Fathers' attendance for family appointments. *Journal of Family Therapy, 23*(1): 3–20.

Watzlawick, P., Jackson, D., & Beavin, J. (1967). *Pragmatics of Human Communication*. New York: Norton.

Watzlawick, P., Weakland, J. H., & Fisch, R. (1974). *Change: The Principles of Problem Formation and Problem Resolution*. New York: Norton.

Weakland, J., Fisch, R., Watzlawick, P., & Bodin, A. (1974). *Brief Therapy: Focused Problem Resolution*. Palo Alto, CA: Norton.

Weerasekera, P. (1996). *Multiperspective Case Formulation*. Florida: Krieger Publishing.

Werner-Wilson, R., Price, S., Zimmerman, T., & Murphy, M. (1997). Client gender as a process variable in marriage and family therapy: Are women clients interrupted more than men clients? *Journal of Family Psychology, 11*: 373–377.

West, C., & Zimmerman, D. (1977). Small insults: A study of interruptions in cross-sex conversations between unacquainted persons. In: B. Thorne, C. Kramarae, & N. Henley (Eds.), *Language, Gender and Society*. Rowley, MA: Newbury House.

White, M. (1987). Anorexia nervosa: A cybernetic approach. In: J. Harkaway (Ed.), *The Family Therapy Collection*. Rockville, MD: Aspen Systems Corporation.

White, M. (1989). The externalizing of the problem and the re-authoring of lives and relationships. In: M. White (Ed.), *Selected Papers*. Adelaide: Dulwich Centre Publications.

White, M. (1995). *Re-authoring Lives: Interviews and Essays* (pp. 3–21). Adelaide: Dulwich Centre Publications.

White, M. (1997). *Narratives of Therapists' Lives*. Adelaide: Dulwich Centre Publications.

White, M., & Epston, D. (1990). *Narrative Means to Therapeutic Ends*. London: Norton.

Williams, J., & Watson, G. (1988). Sexual inequality, family life and family therapy. In: E. Street & W. Dryden (Eds.), *Family Therapy in Britain*. Milton Keynes: Open University Press.

Williams, J., & Watson, G. (1994). Mental health services that empower women: The challenge to clinical psychology. *Clinical Psychology Forum, 64*: 6–12, 291–311.

Winnicott, D. (1971). *Therapeutic Consultations in Child Psychiatry*. London: Hogarth Press and Institute of Psychoanalysis.

Wittgenstein, L. (1951). *Tractatus: Logico-Philosophicus*. New York: Hamilton Press.

Wynne, L., McDaniel, S., & Weber, T. (1986). *Systems Consultation: A New Perspective for Family Therapy*. New York: Guilford Press.

Zimmerman, J., & Dickerson, V. (1993). Separating couples from restraining patterns and the relationship discourse that supports them. *Journal of Marital and Family Therapy, 19*(4): 403–413.

INDEX

Note: For systemic therapy techniques, see entries under *systemic*